Save Your Life

With the Dynamic Duo

D$_3$ and K$_2$

Becoming pH Balanced in an Unbalanced World

Blythe Ayne, Ph.D.

Save Your Life

With the Dynamic Duo

D$_3$ and K$_2$

Becoming pH Balanced in an Unbalanced World

Blythe Ayne, Ph.D.

Save Your Life
With the Dynamic Duo – D3 and K2
Becoming Balanced in an Unbalanced World
Blythe Ayne, Ph.D.

Emerson & Tilman, Publishers
129 Pendleton Way #55
Washougal, WA 98671

Book & cover design by Blythe Ayne
All Text © Blythe Ayne
Graphics: With Gratitude Pixabay Artists:
Kellepic, The Digital Artist, Geralt, Biancamentil, Kahll,
Enrique Lopez Garre, J. Plenio, Alain Audet, WikiImages

Other books in the ***How to Save Your Life*** series:
Save Your Life wiwth the Power of pH Balance
Save Your Life with the Phenomenal Lemon (& Lime!)
Save Your Life with the Elixir of Water
Save Your Life with Stupendous Spices

www.BlytheAyne.com

Save Your Life with with the Dynamic Duo D3 and K2
Becoming Balanced in an Unbalanced World

ebook ISBN: 978-1-947151-79-6
Paperback ISBN: 978-1-947151-80-2
Large Print ISBN: 978-1-947151-81-9
Hardback ISBN: 978-1-947151-82-6

[1. HEALTH & FITNESS/Diet & Nutrition/Nutrition
2. HEALTH & FITNESS/Healing
3. HEALTH & FITNESS/Diseases/General]
BIC: FM
Second Edition

Table of Contents

With gratitude to C. Greear for her editorial assistance.

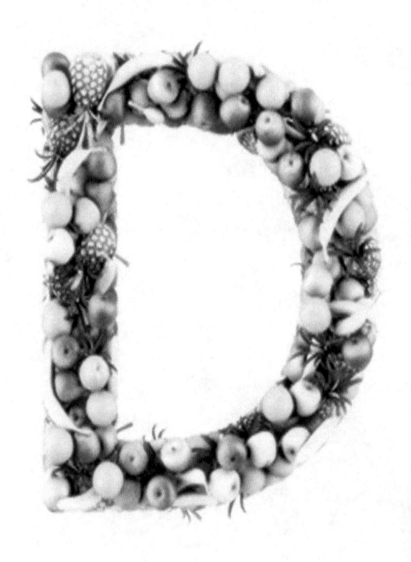

Chapter One

Your Best Defense

The single best defense against all disease—including pandemics—is to have the most well-armored and strongest immune system you can possibly maintain. There are numerous positive contributors to your healthy immunity, but let's take a deeper look at, specifically, D3 and K2.

Vitamin D is Not a Vitamin!

First of all, let's clear up the misnomer of calling D a "vitamin." It's not a vitamin. It's a steroid hormone that controls or affects thousands of genes that are employed in remodeling your tissues, and in sustaining your immune system for optimum health.

So, why is vitamin D called vitamin D? Because, simply, it was discovered after vitamin C. Simple facts are sometimes the strangest. And it was believed at that time to be a nutrient derived from food, not made in the body. And so, its name remains to this day "vitamin D." In humans, the most important compounds in this group are vitamin D3, known as cholecalciferol, and vitamin D2, ergocalciferol.

What, then, _is_ a Vitamin?
Vitamins are organic compounds that are required in our diet because our bodies cannot make them.

Children of the Sun
However, our bodies can and do make the steroid hormone D3 when the sun hits our skin. Amazing, yes?

It wasn't until the following interesting turn of events that it was realized that vitamin D is not a vitamin. In the early 1900s, dogs that lived strictly indoors developed rickets. But eventually, it was noted that dogs raised outside did not develop rickets, and thus did not need the supplement.

Then came the profound aha! that bodies produced the steroid hormone that had come to be known as Vitamin D, on their own when exposed to sunlight— or, for that matter, when exposed to artificial UV light.

The Concept of Vitamins

The idea of vitamins was formulated by Casimir Funk in 1912, a brilliant Polish biochemist who originated the concept of 'vital amines,' i.e., vitamins, present in food and required for health and even survival.

Casimir Funk, with his professional peer, Harry Dubin, created the first vitamin supplement, which they named "Oscodal." Derived from cod liver oil, it contained vitamins A and D. Dr. Funk's comprehension of 'life-giving amines' was absolutely revolutionary in 1912—and has subsequently changed the world!

The Wonders of D3

Although there was an understanding that sunlight and artificial UV light not only prevented but cured rickets, and although Casimir Funk developed a vitamin A and D pill, it wasn't until 1932 that Dr. Askew (cool name!) and Dr. Windaus isolated vitamin D2 from a UV irradiated mixture of ergosterol (a steroid on the cell membranes of fungi)—a plant-based form of vitamin D.

And Vitamin D3 – an animal-based form of vitamin D, was not specifically identified until 1937 by Dr. Windaus and Dr. Bock, when they isolated 7-dehydrocholesterol in hog skin. Hey, you can't make this stuff up. Well, I could, but the facts are more entertaining.

"Daily supplementation with vitamin D results in less severe respiratory infections and less antibiotic use in a susceptible population."
The BMJ (British Medical Journal)

Steroid Superfamily

Vitamin D belongs to the "superfamily" of steroid/ thyroid hormone receptors. As mentioned, vitamin D3 is the natural form of vitamin D in your skin when it's exposed to UV irradiation of 7-dehydrocholesterol—the compound in skin that enables us to manufacture D3.

Cholecalciferol (D3) is converted in the liver to calcifediol, then further converted to calcitriol by the kidneys. Calcitriol circulates as a hormone in your blood, with the life-thriving duties of:
• Regulating the concentration of calcium, magnesium, and phosphate
• Promoting the healthy growth and remodeling of your bones
• Supporting neuromuscular and immune functions
• Regulating cell growth
• Reducing inflammation

This active vitamin D metabolite, calcitriol, binds to the vitamin D receptor in the nuclei of target cells, which allows it to modulate the gene activity of the proteins involved in calcium absorption in the intestine.

Vitamin D receptors maintain skeletal calcium balance with the assistance of the parathyroid hormone, which sustains serum calcium levels. The Vitamin D receptors thus maintain the calcitonin in your bones, intestines, and kidneys, and the calcium and phosphorus levels in your blood, while preserving bone content by, as mentioned, promoting calcium absorption in the intestines, and bone resorption.

Vitamin D receptors also regulate cell proliferation and differentiation, along with having a vital and complex role in supporting the immune system.

Vitamin D receptors are found in your white blood cells, including:

• Monocytes, which influence the process of adaptive immunity

• Activated T cells—lymphocytes in the thymus gland playing a significant role in immune response

• B cells—a part of the adaptive immune system that secretes antibodies and cytokines and presents antigens.

Cytokines act through cell surface receptors, modulating the balance between humoral (body fluids), and cell immune responses.

Furthermore, Vitamin D is directly related to muscle strength, mass, and function.

"As more and more Vitamin D facts
are being discovered in research,
Vitamin D therapy is found to be
imperative to our good health,

> essential for everything from bone
> health, to colds and flu, to heart
> disease, to anti-aging, to many
> types of cancer."
> *Kerry Knox, R.N.*

Relative to sun exposure, diet is a poor source of vitamin D, providing only 40–400 IU per food serving, whereas whole-body UVB exposure for 30 min for a light-skinned person during the summer months will produce upwards of 20,000 IU of vitamin D.

However, UVB exposure and vitamin D production through the skin are reduced with increased skin pigmentation, age, use of sunscreen, and environmental factors such as winter season, high latitude, pollution, cloud cover, and ozone levels.

For instance, sun exposure during most of the winter at latitudes above 33° North (Atlanta, GA, U.S.; Casablanca, Morocco) and below 33 degrees South (Santiago, Chile; New South Wales, Australia; Southern Cape of Africa) provides minimal, if any, vitamin D production.

Get Your D3 Tested
It's a simple blood test called 25-hydroxyvitamin D. The measurement is in nanograms per milliliter. A result below 20 nanograms is too low.

"Vitamin D should be a required 'standard of care' for nearly every serious illness. It improves the immune system, it improves mood, and protects the bones from the demineralization that occurs with dialysis, chemotherapy, steroids and immobility."
www.easy-immune-health.com/vitamin-d-therapy

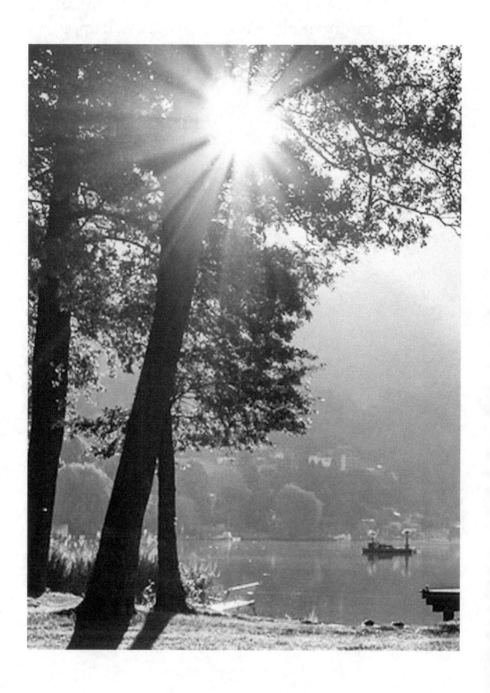

Chapter Two

D3 and Disease

*A*ll well and good, you say, but how does that apply, for example, to a pandemic?

Like this: our bodies make vitamin D3 when the sun hits our skin. But the farther away from the equator one lives, the less—and less!—sun one gets. It gets worse as the days grow short. Therefore, it would be logical to take a D3 supplement to sustain the levels necessary for D3 to fully function and to maintain your good health.

> "It's estimated that up to 75 percent of the population is deficient in Vitamin D, and researchers state that the 400—600 IU's per day recommended by governments is "woefully inadequate."
> *Kerri Knox, RN*

The positive effects of vitamin D3, or, conversely, the negative effects of a deficiency of D3, are profound. Following, you will see a bit of information on a variety of diseases. Not all, by any means, but included are some of the most common diseases, others that have had interesting and promising vitamin D studies, and a few that have had little vitamin D attention.

But they all call for more studies, experiments, and simply, objective, scientific, attention, without anyone's agenda, other than healing the human family.

Please note that there is a glossary and an extensive list of references at the back of the book to help with some of the medical jargon, and references where you can learn more about the topics of your particular interest.

Allergies

Many people with allergies have low D3. Attention parents with children who have a peanut allergy.

Scientific evidence shows that anaphylaxis to various triggers (such as foods, medicines, and insect stings) occurs at much higher rates in areas with less sun exposure.

In addition, asthma, eczema, and atopy (genetic tendency to develop allergic diseases) have been associated with low vitamin D3 levels, particularly for people who have mutations in their vitamin D receptor genes.

Vitamin D3 supplementation given to pregnant women significantly reduced the occurrence of asthma and other allergic diseases in young children.

Alzheimer's Disease

Low serum vitamin D concentrations are associated with prevalent Alzheimer's disease (AD), dementia, and cognitive impairment. Given the high rates of vitamin D deficiency in older adults and continued uncertainty about the causes of AD and other forms of dementia, this is problematic.

Both the 1,25-dihydroxy vitamin D3 receptor and 1α-hydroxylase, the enzyme responsible for synthesizing the bioactive form of vitamin D, are found throughout the human brain. In a healthy brain, vitamin D increases the phagocytic clearance of amyloid plaques by stimulating macrophages, and reduces amyloid-induced cytotoxicity and apoptosis in primary cortical neurons.

Vitamin D deficiency has been linked to vascular dysfunction and stroke, as well as brain atrophy, although reverse causation (the opposite) is also possible, due to the onset of dementia, which may lead to poor dietary habits and reduced outdoor activity.

Participants in a study were followed for five-and-a-half years. During which time, 171 participants developed all-cause dementia, and 102 developed

Alzheimer's disease. The risk of developing both all-cause dementia and AD was significantly higher in participants who were either vitamin D deficient, or severely deficient.

Those who were deficient had about a 51 percent increased risk of all-cause dementia, whereas the increased risk for those who were severely deficient was 122 percent.

The strength of the association for incident AD was similar to that observed for all-cause dementia. The risk of all-cause dementia and AD markedly increases at D3 concentrations below 50 nanomoles per liter.

Anorexia Nervosa

Anorectics have low D3. And, interestingly, anorexia is notably higher among people born in March!

A study found that Vitamin D deficiency is significantly prevalent in teens who have an eating disorder, which increases the risk for osteoporosis, cessation of estrogen, and increased cortisol levels, all of which contribute to bone loss.

A study in Israel found that participants in their early to late teens who had anorexia, bulimia, and binge eating, had vitamin D levels and bone mineral density lower than 32 nanograms per milliliter, the level where bone growth is maintained. It was also found that the lumbar spine bone mineral density was low.

Arthritis and Bone and Joint Issues

Studies show that as much as 80 percent of people with arthritis and/or bone and joint issues are vitamin D3 deficient.

Vitamin D plays a significant role in joint health—low levels increase the risk of rheumatologic conditions such as arthritis. Several studies have found low blood levels of vitamin D in patients with osteoarthritis of the hip and knee.

In another study of more than 2,000 people, researchers found that vitamin D deficiency was strongly associated with disabling symptoms for people with rheumatoid arthritis.

Vitamin D deficiency interferes with immune tolerance, causing the development of autoimmune diseases such as rheumatoid arthritis (RA), while adequate vitamin D supports immune tolerance.

Vitamin D acts on the immune system both in an endocrine (cells release hormones that act on distant target cells) and in a paracrine (cells act on nearby cells) manner. It regulates the immune response by:
- Decreasing antigen presentation
- Inhibiting pro-inflammatory T helper type 1cells
- Inducing regulatory T cells

These data contribute to clarifying the development and progression of autoimmune inflammatory conditions in general, and rheumatoid arthritis in particular, when vitamin D is deficient.

Data from animal studies indicate that the D3 metabolite (a small molecule involved in metabolism) and its analog suppress collagen-induced arthritis, while vitamin D receptor agonists (a substance which initiates a physiological response when combined with a receptor) also prevent and suppress established collagen-induced arthritis.

In addition, there is data showing that vitamin D3 may decrease due to inflammation in active rheumatoid arthritis. Supplementation with vitamin D is necessary, in order to maintain immune function and prevent the development of autoimmune diseases.

> "It's now known that every cell and tissue within the body has a vitamin D protein receptor."
> *Jeff T. Bowles*

Asthma

Asthma has been on the rise, especially since the 1980s. Asthma affects 300 million children and adults around the world, and is one of the biggest health burdens, with the number rising every year.

Prof. Martineau and colleagues of Queen Mary University of London, reviewed seven studies of 955 subjects with asthma that investigated the effects of vitamin D supplementation on disease severity. The researchers found that vitamin D supplementation reduced asthma-related emergency visits and hospital admissions by 50 percent as compared with a placebo.

Also, vitamin D3 supplements reduced the need for steroid tablets or injections by 30 percent among adults who experience an asthma attack. The researchers found that patients whose vitamin D3 levels were low at the outset of the study experienced the greatest benefit from vitamin D3 supplements, with their need for treatment with steroid tablets or injections falling by 55 percent.

Further, increased intake of vitamin D during pregnancy has proven to have a positive influence on asthma in both children and adults.

A survey of 75 Italian asthmatic children revealed that their vitamin D-deficiency was 53.3 percent. In a North American survey, 17 percent of asthmatics had vitamin D deficiency, with a positive correlation observed between vitamin D3 levels and lung function. Another study revealed that low serum vitamin D3 levels in children at the age of six years predicted asthma-associated symptoms by the time they were 14 years old.

A. Gupta, and colleagues were the pioneer researchers in observing that serum vitamin D levels were found to be lowest among children with steroid-resistant asthma (STRA), with reduced lung function and increased corticosteroid use. Low vitamin D3 levels increase the airway's smooth muscle (ASM) and reduce lung function in severe asthma.

A 4-year study by Brehm and colleagues established a causal relationship between serum vitamin D levels and asthma exacerbations in 1,024 North American asthmatic children. This study confirmed that levels of vitamin D below 30 nanograms per milliliter had increased risk of asthma exacerbations.

Another study conducted on 560 Puerto Rican children, ages 6 to 14 years of age with asthma, reported that children with vitamin D3 insufficiency were 2.6 times more at risk of developing asthma exacerbations.

A study conducted on 70 adult asthmatic patients and 20 controls concluded that serum vitamin D level was significantly decreased in asthmatic patients—19.88 nanograms per milliliter, as compared to the control group—33.5 nanograms per milliliter.

A study consisting of 100 asthmatic children revealed that monthly doses of 60,000 IU of vitamin D3 significantly decreased the number of asthma exacerbations and reduced the use of steroids and emergency hospital visits.

Autism

Autism has had a shocking increase in recent years, with autistic births peaking during the months of November and March (it's been suggested that the sun reflecting off snow has a D3 generating effect on December through February births). Additionally, some of the genes involved in autism are also involved in ADD/ADHD, and thus D3 treatment may be extremely beneficial in those disorders, as well.

Mounting evidence points to the possibility that gestational and early childhood vitamin D deficiency cause some cases of autism. Vitamin D is a neurosteroid, active in brain development, with effects on cellular proliferation and differentiation, neurotrophic and neuroprotective actions, calcium signaling, neurotransmission, and synaptic plasticity.

Children who are, or who will become, autistic have lower vitamin D levels at 3 months during gestation, at birth, and at age 8, than their siblings.

Two trials found that high dose vitamin D improves the symptoms of autism in 75 percent of autistic children—some of the improvements were remarkable.

In the first study, vitamin D doses were 300 IU per kilogram of weight, per day, up to a maximum of 5000 IU per day. The highest final vitamin D level reached was 45 nanograms per milliliter. In the other study, the dose was 150,000 IU per month, plus 400 IU per day, which resulted in the highest final D3 level being 52 nanograms per milliliter.

Yet another study showed that vitamin D3 supplementation of 5,000 IU per day during pregnancy, and 1,000 IU per day for the children during infancy and early childhood, reduced the expected incidence of autism with mothers who already had one autistic child from 20 percent to 5 percent!

Given those facts, practitioners might consider treating pregnant and lactating women with 5,000 IU of D3 per day, and infants and young children with 150 IU per kg per day, checking the D3 levels every 3 months. These doses have proven to increase the 25(OH)D blood levels to those recommended by the Endocrine Society.

Bone Spurs

There are many reports of bone spurs disappearing with people on high doses of D3. Jeff Bowles, Author of The Miraculous Cure for and Prevention of All Diseases, tells of a bone spur he had on his elbow for years that disappeared in nine months of high-dose vitamin D3.

He further tells of a man who had two bone spurs on his ankles that his foot doctor said were the largest he'd ever seen, that he'd had for 20 years, and they were gone after a few months of 26,000 IU D3 per day.

Cancer

In 1941 Frank Apperly, an American pathologist, published data that demonstrated for the first time the inverse correlation between the levels of ultra-violet (UV) radiation and the mortality rates from cancers in North America.

Apperly observed that "The presence of skin cancer was really only an occasional accompaniment of relative cancer immunity, but the immunity was related to exposure to ultraviolet radiation ... A closer study of the action of solar radiation on the body might well reveal the nature of cancer immunity."

Since Apperly's observations, it has been confirmed that there is an increased risk of dying of various cancers at latitudes further from the equator. In addition, it has been demonstrated that sun exposure results in favorable prognosis and increased survival rate in various malignancies, including malignant melanoma. Lab results show the importance of the vitamin D hormone and receptor systems when studying the pathogenesis and progression of cancer, supporting the hypothesis that vitamin D is linked to cancer prevention.

Inadequate sunlight leads to more than increased bone disease and cancer, including decreased protection against infectious disease. It has been demonstrated that D is a direct regulator of the anti-microbial innate immune response, which, in mammals, provides a rapid response to repel assaults from numerous infectious agents including bacteria, viruses, fungi, and parasites. (Wang 2004)

A PubMed database of 63 studies of vitamin D in relation to cancer risk, including colon, breast, prostate, and ovarian cancer, showed a clear relationship between sufficient vitamin D and lower risk of cancer. Improving vitamin D status with vitamin D supplementation can reduce cancer incidence and mortality at low cost.

GrassrootsHealth found an inverse association between vitamin D serum levels and all non-skin cancer incidence. Those with vitamin D serum levels greater than 40 nanograms per milliliter, had a 67 percent lower risk of cancer when compared with those less than 20 nanograms per milliliter.

In the midst of all of this human suffering that can so readily be improved, drug companies are putting their figurative heads together to discover ways to separate the components of Vitamin D to take the anticancer element and put it in a patented drug to treat cancer. Then they can charge us for it, which they can't do now when we can go to the store and buy our own D-supplement-cancer-preventative.

Doctors and researchers who have been in the trenches with cancer for years and decades, past and present, address the importance of D3 without the least ambiguity. Read on....

"Using newly available data on worldwide cancer incidence, researchers have shown a clear association between deficiency in exposure to sunlight and endometrial cancer, kidney cancer, ovarian cancer, and lung cancer."

Science Daily

"There have been over 3,000 studies showing the relationship between vitamin D and cancer."

www.easy-immune-health.com/Vitamin-D-and-Cancer

"Those who have attempted to convince the world that the sun, the earth's primary source of energy and life, causes cancer, have done so with malicious intent to deceive the masses into retreating from the one thing that can prevent disease."

Dr. Dave Mihalovic

Oliver Gillie has been trying to get the UK to increase their woefully inadequate minimum requirements of Vitamin D3, to no avail. He is quoted as saying, "Indeed, it may be that insufficient vitamin D is a risk factor for most, if not all, types of cancer."

Oliver Gillie
Author of Scotland's Health Deficit,
an Explanation and a Plan and
Sunlight Robbery

"Despite the fact that researchers are adamant that Vitamin D plays a pivotal role in cancer prevention, The American Cancer Society has taken the official stance that people should not take vitamins to prevent cancer."

Samuel Epstein MD
Author of: American Cancer Society –
More Interested in Accumulating Wealth
Than Saving Lives

"If we take in enough vitamin D to control our genes in such a way that we're less likely to get cancer, (we'll also be) less likely to suffer a lot of age-related problems."

Bill Falloon, MD Founder of the Life Extension Foundation

"Taking a daily 10- to 15-minute walk in the sun not only clears your head, relieves stress, and increases circulation—it could also cut your risk of breast cancer in half."

Dr. Esther John

"The majority of Americans, including many doctors, have been tricked into believing that the sun is somehow toxic, a carcinogen, and an overall deadly health hazard that should be avoided at all costs. How wrong we are! The sun, instead of causing cancer, prevents cancer, and can be even used to treat cancer."

Dr. Mark Sircus

"Paradoxically, outdoor workers have a decreased risk of melanoma compared with indoor workers, suggesting that chronic sunlight exposure can have a protective effect."

The Lancet

Although Vitamin D deficiency is known mainly for its association with fractures and bone disease, its newly recognized association with risk of several types of cancer is receiving considerable attention. The high prevalence of vitamin D deficiency, combined with the discovery of increased risks of certain types of cancer in those who are deficient, indicate that vitamin D deficiency accounts for thousands of premature deaths from colon, breast, ovarian, and prostate cancer annually.

American Public Health

"Low levels of vitamin D is connected to the more aggressive forms of prostate cancer. Eighty-seven men in this study had aggressive prostate cancer, and had a median level of 22.7 nanograms per milliliter of vitamin D, significantly below the normal level of more than 30 nanograms per milliliter.

"Men with dark skin, low levels of vitamin D intake, (and/or) low sun exposure should be tested for vitamin D deficiency when diagnosed with an elevated PSA or prostate cancer. Then the deficiency should be corrected with supplements."

Dr. Adam Murphy
Clinical Oncology

"The sun protects us from breast cancer, colon cancer, ovarian cancer, and prostate cancer. It can also prevent heart disease, high blood pressure, osteoporosis, psoriasis, MS, diabetes, and seasonal affective disorder. Cancer is actually helped by sunbathing. Persons who receive the most sunlight have less cancer."

Dr. Richard Hobday, The Healing Sun

"Vitamin D levels of 48 nanograms per milliliter or higher were linked to a 67 percent reduction in cancer risk when compared to those whose levels were 20 nanograms per milliliter or less."

UC San Diego

"(Since) more than 2,000 genes are modulated by D3 we can begin to understand why vitamin D is important in cancer treatment."

Dr. Mark Sircus

"In our study, we discovered that for every 10 nanograms per milliliter increase in a woman's vitamin D blood level, the relative risk of cancer dropped by 35 percent."

Dr. Joan Lappe

Cartilage Degeneration

A woman told by her doctors that she needed both of her knees replaced started taking 2,000 IU D3 for two months, then raised it to 10,000 for the third month, and her knees healed.

Gabby Joseph (University of California, San Francisco) and colleagues found a significant inverse association between dietary vitamin D intake and cartilage degeneration among 1,785 patients.

Higher vitamin D intake was significantly associated with a reduction in cartilage Whole-Organ Magnetic Resonance score (WORMS), where lower scores indicate less degeneration. Daily vitamin D supplementation was significantly associated with a lower cartilage WORMS score in the medial femur.

The researchers also demonstrated a longitudinal association between vitamin D supplementation and reduced joint degeneration over four years of follow-up among individuals who took supplements consistently, with 300 IU taken at least 4–6 days per week being the smallest dose and lowest frequency to show an inverse association with WORMS progression.

The test showed that taking at least 400 IU of vitamin D on at least 1–3 days per week was associated with a significantly reduced risk for cartilage, meniscus, and bone marrow Whole-Organ Magnetic Resonance score worsening over four years, while taking 400 IU on at least 4–6 days per week was associated with significantly reduced odds of joint structure degeneration.

Vitamin D deficiency negatively impacts the pathogenesis of cartilage degeneration in osteoarthritis (OA), directly through its influence on extracellular matrix activity, and indirectly through its negative effects on bone metabolism.

Cavities

Dr. Cannel, head of the Vitamin D Institute, cited that giving children 1,000 IU D3 per day stopped the formation of cavities.

There has been considerable evidence of a relationship between vitamin D deficiency and cavities, for decades. Many studies were conducted in the 1930s and 1940s that supplementing children with vitamin D would prevent cavities. As previously mentioned, up to 20,000 IU of vitamin D3 can be obtained by sitting in the sun for half-an-hour in the middle of the day.

Schroth and colleagues ran a study evaluating the relationship between vitamin D levels and dental caries in Canadian school students, with a total of 1,017 children, aged 6 to 11 years, included in the study. It was observed that 56.4 percent of the children had caries, which was associated with vitamin D3 levels below 30 nanograms per milliliter.

The results suggest that failure to achieve the optimum vitamin D levels is associated with the likelihood of dental caries being increased by 39 percent.

Chronic Pain

Studies investigating the relationship between vitamin D3 deficiency and chronic pain are multitudinous and varied. Here are a few examples: Eight patients with tension headaches, fatigue, pain in the low back, hip, and lower extremities, all had D3 levels of less than 10 nanograms per milliliter. The pain medications they were taking had no effect on their pain.

They were treated with 1,000 to 1,500 IU of D3 daily (author note: low dose), with complete resolution of their headaches in 4 to 8 weeks. After three months, their vitamin D levels had stabilized in normal range and their other symptoms had a markedly declined.

Six patients with severe back pain and one patient with persistent back pain following failed back surgery were treated with 1,000 to 4,000 IU of cholecalciferol daily, with the results of improvement, to complete resolution, of pain within 3 to 6 weeks.

A 16-year-old girl with sickle cell disease had chronic pain, throbbing headaches, nausea, and epigastric pain, all of which were unaffected by nonsteroidal anti-inflammatory drugs (NSAIDs), oral opioids, or other multidisciplinary pain management strategies. Her vitamin D level was 7.9 nanograms per milliliter. She was treated with 50,000 IU vitamin D twice per week. By three-and-a-half months her serum vitamin D3 was 30 nanograms per milliliter, and all her pain symptoms were gone.

An elderly woman complaining of persistent around-the-clock muscular pain had vitamin D3 level of 15 nanograms per milliliter. After being treated with 50,000 IU of ergocalciferol (D2—generally not preferred!) for 8 weeks, she experienced a significant decline in her symptoms.

Several patients believed to have a metastatic malignancy underwent imaging and laboratory studies. They were found, instead, to have vitamin D deficiency. Adequate vitamin D resulted in symptom resolution.

Two patients, one who had gastric bypass surgery, and the other who had jejunoileal bypass surgery, complained of fatigue, muscle aches, bone pain, and muscle weakness. They were both found to be deficient in vitamin D. Adequate vitamin D over time resulted in symptom resolution.

The redundant refrain: there need to be more studies around the amazing effect of vitamin D3 on chronic pain.

Colds and Flu

Examples of the positive effect of vitamin D on the common cold and the flu are numerous. Here's one: At Winthrop University Hospital, Mineola, New York, supplements of vitamin D given to a group of volunteers reduced their episodes of infection with colds and flu by 70 percent over three years.

COPD

Chronic obstructive pulmonary disease, or COPD, includes a number of lung conditions such as emphysema and chronic bronchitis. COPD deaths are generally due to a sudden worsening of symptoms, often triggered by viral upper respiratory infections.

Data were analyzed from 469 COPD patients from three clinical trials, which took place in the United Kingdom, Belgium, and the Netherlands. Taking vitamin D3 supplements was associated with a 45 percent reduction in lung attacks among patients who were deficient in vitamin D, although there was no reduction among patients with higher vitamin D levels. (Author's note: Their levels are not provided. Perhaps they were still low.)

"Vitamin D supplementation is safe and inexpensive. This is a potentially highly cost-effective treatment that could be targeted at those who have low vitamin D levels following routine testing. A fifth of COPD patients in the UK, about 240,000 people, have low levels of vitamin D," Dr. Martineau, the author of the study, said.

Worldwide, more than 170 million people have COPD, which caused an estimated 3.2 million deaths in 2015.

Covid-19

Here are a few of the following terms in a short glossary, which I hope will be helpful:

25-hydroxyvitamin D (25(OH)D) – This is, simply: Vitamin D3.

Cathelicidins – small, cationic, positively charged ions, that are antimicrobial peptides (compounds consisting of two or more amino acids linked in a chain), found in humans and other species. These proteolytically (proteins broken down into simpler compounds) activated peptides are part of the innate immune system of many vertebrates. Cathelicidins serve a critical role in your immune defense against invasive bacterial infection. The cathelicidin family of antimicrobial peptides (AMPs) also includes the defensins.

Defensins are small cysteine-rich cationic proteins across, found in vertebrate and invertebrate animals, plants, and fungi. They are host defense peptides, displaying direct antimicrobial activity or immune signaling activities, or both.

Macrophage – a large white blood cell that is an important part of our immune system that 'eats' bacteria, viruses, fungi, and parasites. They are born from white blood cells called monocytes, produced by stem cells in our bone marrow.

Aldosterone – a corticosteroid hormone (hormones produced in the adrenal cortex) which stimulates absorption of sodium by the kidneys, regulating water and salt balance.

Angiotensin – a protein that promotes aldosterone secretion, which tends to raise blood pressure.

Renin-angiotensin system (RAS) – a hormone system that regulates blood pressure and fluid and electrolyte balance, as well as systemic vascular resistance – blood pressure and blood flow.

Proinflammatory cytokines – produced predominantly by activated macrophages, involved in the up-regulation of inflammatory reactions.

*   *   *

The following article reviews the roles of vitamin D in reducing the risk of respiratory infections, and provides a thumbnail sketch of the epidemiology of COVID-19.

Vitamin D helps reduce the risk of infections by inducing cathelicidins and defensins to lower viral replication rates, and reducing concentrations of pro-inflammatory cytokines that produce the inflammation that injures the lining of the lungs, which leads to pneumonia, as well as increasing concentrations of anti-inflammatory cytokines.

Evidence supporting the idea that vitamin D3 has the potential to be effective in reducing the risk of

COVID-19 infection includes these facts:

• The initial outbreak occurred in winter, when 25-hydroxyvitamin D (25(OH)D) (Vitamin D3) concentrations are lowest

• The number of cases in the Southern Hemisphere, where it was summer was lower than in the Northern Hemisphere, coming out of winter

• Vitamin D deficiency has been found to contribute to acute respiratory distress syndrome (ARDS)

• Fatality rates increase with age and/or chronic disease comorbidity (the simultaneous presence of two chronic diseases)

• Both of which are associated with lower vitamin D3 concentration

To reduce the risk of infection, the NCBI article recommends that people take 10,000 IU per day of vitamin D3 for a few weeks to rapidly raise their immune system.

"Your goal is to raise your 25(OH)D concentrations to 40-60 nanograms per milliliter (100-150 nanomoles per liter). For treatment of people who become infected with COVID-19, higher vitamin D3 doses are useful. Randomized controlled trials and large population studies are urgently needed to support and/or refine these recommendations."

https://www.ncbi.nlm.nih.gov/pubmed/32252338

Research demonstrates that the SARS-Cov-2 virus (Covid-19) enters cells via the angiotensin-converting enzyme 2 (ACE2). When the coronavirus replicates it suppresses ACE2, impairing the hormone system that regulates blood pressure, blood flow, and electrolyte balance. This creates what is referred to as a "cytokine storm" where the body mounts all its resources to attack itself, causing acute respiratory distress syndrome (ARDS).

To anthropomorphize this scene, the virus cleverly invades a territory (a human body), strategically places bombs that, when they go off, makes the natives think all their peers are enemies, and they wipe each other out. Then the virus sits back, waiting until another "territory" comes along to invade.

Vitamin D3 to the rescue! It balances the renin-angiotensin system—RAS, (the hormone system that regulates blood pressure, blood flow, and electrolyte balance) and reduces lung damage.

Vitamin D supplementation has been shown to increase immunity, reduce inflammation, and reduce the risk of acute respiratory tract infections. It's considered safe to take oral vitamin D supplements at doses up to 250 mcg (10,000 IU) per day.

Chronic hypovitaminosis D (insufficient Vitamin D) induces pulmonary fibrosis through the activation of RAS, and has been strongly associated with acute respiratory distress syndrome (ARDS), as well as with various comorbidities associated with deaths during SARS-Cov-2 infections.

Diabetes

Diabetes occurs when insulin is destroyed by the immune system. A recent study has shown that high doses of vitamin D3 stops Type 1 diabetes in its tracks. Might it be as effective for Type 2 diabetes?

The International Diabetes Federation estimates the number of people with diabetes to be nearly 285 million, or 7 percent of the world's population, which is expected to exceed 435 million by 2030. In the United States alone, an estimated 79 million people are pre-diabetic.

There is growing evidence that vitamin D deficiency could be a contributing factor in the development of both type 1 and type 2 diabetes. The beta cell in the pancreas that secretes insulin has been shown to contain vitamin D receptors (VDR), while vitamin D3 treatment improves glucose tolerance and insulin resistance.

Vitamin D3 deficiency leads to reduced insulin secretion, while supplementation with vitamin D3 has been shown to restore insulin secretion in animals. Researchers have also found an indirect effect on insulin secretion, potentially by a calcium effect on insulin secretion.

Vitamin D contributes to normalizing extracellular calcium, which assures normal calcium flux through cell membranes. Thus, it seems probable that low vitamin D would diminish calcium's ability to affect insulin secretion.

Other relationships between adequate vitamin D and diabetes include improving insulin action by stimulating the expression of the insulin receptor, and enhancing insulin responsiveness for glucose transport. This would have an indirect effect on insulin via calcium's action on insulin secretion, thus reducing systemic inflammation.

Vitamin D and Type 2 Diabetes

After a meta-analysis of the impact of vitamin D and calcium on glycemic control in patients with type 2 diabetes, it was concluded that insufficient vitamin D and calcium hinders glycemic control. Supplementing both nutrients may be necessary to optimize glucose metabolism.

The Nurses Health Study that included 83,779 women over 20 years of age found an increased risk of type 2 diabetes in those with low vitamin D. A combined daily intake of more than 800 IU of vitamin D and 1,000 mg of calcium reduced the risk of type 2 diabetes by 33 percent.

The National Health and Nutrition Examination Survey (NHANES), between 1988 and 1994, demonstrated that low vitamin D levels were predictive of the future development of type 2 diabetes. Increasing vitamin D serum levels to normal led to a 55 percent reduction in the risk of developing type 2 diabetes.

The results in a multi-ethnic study of 712 subjects indicated that vitamin D was significantly correlated to insulin resistance and beta cell function, with the conclusion that low vitamin D levels play a significant role in the pathogenesis of type 2 diabetes.

The NHANES group also evaluated 9,773 U.S. adults over 18 years of age, and established a link between serum vitamin D levels, glucose homeostasis, and the evolution of diabetes. Further, it's suggested that patients with elevated A1C levels should be evaluated for vitamin D insufficiency.

Vitamin D and Type 1 Diabetes

Studies suggest that low vitamin D may be associated with an increased risk of type 1 diabetes, as well. There is a greater incidence of type 1 diabetes-related to geographic variation, with locations at higher latitudes having more type 1 diabetes, the probable result of less sunshine, and, therefore, lower levels of vitamin D.

Data were collected during one year on 10,821 children regarding vitamin D3 supplementation and the presence of suspected rickets, as it related to the development of type 1 diabetes in northern Finland. The results were amazing. Children who took 2,000 IU of vitamin D daily were 80 percent less likely to develop type 1 diabetes. It may be crucial for children to take vitamin D supplementation during their first year of life to help avoid the development of type 1 diabetes.

A vitamin D study conducted by Zipitis and colleagues demonstrated that vitamin D3 supplementation in early childhood decreased the risk of developing type 1 diabetes by 29 percent, compared to children who were not given vitamin D3 supplements. And, again, starting vitamin D3 supplements soon after birth may be a protective strategy against the development of type 1 diabetes.

Dr. Gregory and colleagues suggested that pregnant women and nursing mothers take vitamin D3 supplements to make sure their serum levels are optimal. This research showed that adequate vitamin D status in mothers reduced the development of type 1 diabetes in their children. Because vitamin D is a powerful modulator of the immune system and helps regulate cell proliferation and differentiation, once again, it appears that vitamin D can play a role in preventing type 1 diabetes.

Maintaining adequate vitamin D during pregnancy, nursing, infancy, and childhood helps prevent type 1 diabetes, although it is still unknown whether the genetics of type 1 diabetes place individuals at risk for vitamin D deficiency, or whether vitamin D deficiency places individuals at risk for type 1 diabetes.

Fibromyalgia
Fibromyalgia is characterized by chronic, widespread musculoskeletal pain, fatigue, and tenderness in specific, localized areas—trigger points—and is often accompanied by altered sleep, and altered mood.

People with fibromyalgia diagnosis and vitamin D less than 30 nanograms per milliliter were recruited in a study to receive 50,000 IU of oral vitamin D once per week for three months. The participants' vitamin D levels increased significantly after three months from 18.4 nanograms per milliliter to 33.8 nanograms per milliliter, with 72.2 percent of the participants reporting that they experienced a significant improvement in symptoms, including a reduction in the number of painful trigger points after three months.

> "Vitamin D actually prevents the very health problems that it is accused of causing."
> *Robert Barefoot*

Heart Disease

Vitamin D deficiency has been linked to several cardiovascular risk factors. In addition, direct effects of vitamin D upon smooth muscle calcification and proliferation could contribute to its effect on cardiovascular health.

In a study from 1988 to 1994, low vitamin D was associated with cardiovascular disease (CVD) and select CVD risk factors, including diabetes mellitus (DM), obesity, and hypertriglyceridemia.

And in a study between 1993 to 1999 of 18,225 U.S. men, low vitamin D3 was associated with a higher risk of myocardial infarction. A high prevalence of hypovitaminosis D3 was found in individuals with cardiovascular diseases, namely coronary heart disease and heart failure.

In a meta-analysis of 19 prospective studies of 65,994 participants, Dr. Wang and colleagues demonstrated a linear, inverse association between circulating vitamin D and risk of cardiovascular diseases.

Coronary Artery Disease

The association of vitamin D deficiency with coronary artery diseases (CADs) has been investigated in many studies. In 1978, a Danish study found that low vitamin D levels were significantly associated with angina and myocardial infarction.

In a multi-center U.S. study evaluating patients admitted with acute coronary syndrome (ACS), about 95 percent of the patients were found to have low vitamin D levels. In another study conducted by Dr. Dziedziel, low vitamin D levels were observed in patients with myocardial infarction history.

The Health Professionals Follow-up Study, which included 18,225 participants, had similar findings. At a 10-year follow-up, participants with a normal vitamin D level had half the risk of myocardial infarction.

In another large study of 10,170 participants, low vitamin D levels were found to be associated with increased risk of ischemic heart disease, myocardial infarction, and early death during nine years of follow-up. Additionally, in a meta-analysis of 18 studies, low vitamin D levels were related to an increased risk of ischemic heart disease and early death.

Pathophysiology

It's hypothesized that vitamin D deficiency increases blood pressure through the renin-angiotensin system.

In 2011, a study conducted by Argacha and colleagues revealed that vitamin D deficient male rats have increased systolic blood pressure, superoxide anion production, angiotensin II, and atrial natriuretic peptide, with observed changes in fifty-one cardiac gene expressions important in the regulation of oxidative stress and myocardial hypertrophy.

Another study of vitamin D deficient mice showed increased systolic blood pressure, diastolic blood pressure, high plasma renin-angiotensin activity and reduced urinary sodium excretion, which was reversed after a mere 6 weeks of a vitamin D-sufficient diet.

In the same study, vitamin D deficient mice on a high-fat diet had increased atherosclerosis in their aorta with increased macrophage infiltration, fat deposition, and endoplasmic reticulum stress activation. These results indicate vitamin D deficiency is associated with the development of hypertension and accelerated atherosclerosis.

For the first time in humans, a study of 3,316 patients, from 1997 to 2000 in southwest Ludwigshafen, Germany, showed a steady increase of plasma renin concentration, and an increase in angiotensin 2, with declining levels of vitamin D3.

Hypertension

Hypertension is the most common presentation to primary care providers and represents a major chronic health disease in developed countries. The prevalence of hypertension in adults is approximately 29 percent, with an estimated 1.6 billion cases of hypertension expected in 2025.

There is accumulating evidence for the association between vitamin D and blood pressure. An analysis of 12,644 participants over 20 years of age showed an inverse association between vitamin D level and blood pressure.

Forman and colleagues have also demonstrated an inverse association between vitamin D and risk of incident hypertension from two studies including 613 men followed for 4 to 8 years, and 38,388 men followed for 16 to 18 years, from the Health Professionals' Follow-Up Study, and 1,198 women followed for 4 to 8 years, and 77,531 women followed for 16 to 18 years, from The Nurses' Health Study.

In a study of 833 Caucasian males in Uppsala, Sweden, a three times higher prevalence of confirmed hypertension was found in participants with vitamin D levels less than 37.5 nanomoles per liter. Additionally, a cross-sectional analysis of hypertension of 1,460 participants in Shanghai, China showed a high prevalence of vitamin D deficiency (55.8 percent) in middle-aged and elderly Chinese men.

In Peru, a study of 1,441 adolescents aged 13 to 15 showed an inverse association between vitamin D deficiency and blood pressure, which will likely predispose a risk of hypertension in adulthood.

Aging

Older adults are at increased risk for vitamin D deficiency, due to reduced vitamin D intake and decreased synthesis from the sun. Beyond skeletal health, evidence has linked vitamin D deficiency to cardiovascular diseases and hypertension in older patients.

The increased cardiovascular diseases are due to vascular endothelial dysfunction, which is shown by decreased peripheral arterial endothelium-dependent dilatation. The mechanisms underpinning this association have been attributed primarily to reductions in nitric oxide synthesis and increases in oxidative stress.

In a study conducted by Dr. Kestenbaum, 2,312 participants over 65 years of age without cardiovascular disease at baseline, were followed for a median period of 14 years. Their results showed that low 25(OH)D was associated with cardiovascular disease and mortality.

Resistant Hypertension

The prevalence of resistant hypertension almost doubled from 5.5 percent during 1988 to 1994 to 11.8 percent during 2005 to 2008. Low vitamin D was linked to resistant hypertension, only secondary to obesity and excessive adipose tissue, and metabolic disturbances, including insulin resistance. In a study of 150 patients, lower vitamin D level was associated with resistant hypertension.

Cerebrovascular Accident

Cerebrovascular accident (CVA) is a devastating neurological condition, which can cause physical impairment and even death. Accumulating evidence suggests that vitamin D deficiency is associated with an increased risk of CVA. The underlying mechanisms have been largely attributed to the association of vitamin D with cardiovascular risk factors such as hypertension. Epidemiological studies suggest that vitamin D deficiency is an independent risk factor for CVA.

In a study conducted by Dr. Sun and colleagues of 464 subjects, low vitamin D levels were associated with increased risk of developing CVA, and vitamin D deficiency was found to be a risk factor for CVA unrelated to race.

Mortality

A study of 3,258 patients at Cardiac Center, Ludwig-shafen, Germany, with a median follow-up of 7.7 years, showed that low vitamin D level is independently associated with higher all-cause mortality and cardiovascular mortality.

In Finland, a study of 1,136 participants from the Kuopio Ischaemic Heart Disease Risk Factor Study (KIHD), showed that vitamin D deficiency was associated with a higher risk of death.

Vitamin D Supplementation

In a randomization study, Vimaleswaran and colleagues found genetic evidence that increased vitamin D concentrations are associated with reduced blood pressure and the risk of hypertension.

Hypoglycemia

Vitamin D3 is believed to help improve the body's sensitivity to insulin—the hormone responsible for regulating blood sugar levels—and thus reduce the risk of insulin resistance, which is often a precursor to type 2 diabetes. Some scientists also believe D3 may help regulate the production of insulin in the pancreas.

Vitamin D levels below 20 nanograms per milliliter is deficient. However, it is now known that raising the amount of D3 significantly above that threshold to around 60-80 nanograms per milliliter can help keep blood glucose levels under control, which is vital for people with diabetes.

Aids weight loss – studies have shown that good vitamin D status helps to reduce parathyroid hormone (PTH) levels, which in the long-term may promote weight loss and reduce risk of obesity, which is a major risk factor for type 2 diabetes.

Regulates appetite – vitamin D can increase your body's levels of the hormone leptin, which controls body fat storage and triggers the sensation of satiety, giving the feeling of having eaten enough and thus lowering hunger levels.

Reduces belly fat – an increase in vitamin D can help lower levels of cortisol, a stress hormone produced in the adrenal glands. Cortisol is involved in a number of important functions, including the body's response to stress and regulation of blood pressure. But higher and more prolonged levels of the hormone in the blood can lead to increased abdominal fat, which is linked to various health conditions, including diabetes.

Incontinence

Vitamin D3 deficiency appears to contribute to pelvic floor disorders. "Higher vitamin D3 levels were associated with a decreased risk of any pelvic floor disorder in all the women in our study," reported researcher Samuel Badalian, MD, PhD, of SUNY Upstate Medical University in Syracuse, N.Y.

In addition, recent studies have also linked osteoporosis to pelvic floor disorders. A study of vitamin D levels and pelvic floor disorders reported by 1,881 non-pregnant women over 20 years of age showed 82 percent of the women had deficient vitamin D levels.

One or more pelvic floor disorders were reported by 23 percent of the women, and average vitamin D levels were significantly lower among those with at least one pelvic floor disorder or incontinence.

A woman who was on 10,000 IU D3 per day for six months self-reported that it cured her incontinence.

Infertility

Ninety-three percent of infertile women are vitamin D3 deficient! One woman who failed three in vitro fertilization attempts started taking 20,000 IU D3 per day and soon became pregnant.

Kidney Disease

Chronic kidney disease (CKD) is recognized as a significant global health problem due to the increased risk of morbidity and mortality. Vitamin D deficiency or insufficiency is common in patients with CKD, and serum levels of vitamin D appear to have an inverse correlation with kidney function.

Evidence shows that vitamin D deficiency contributes to deteriorating renal function, and increased morbidity and mortality in patients with CKD.

Chronic kidney disease is characterized by a progressive loss of renal function that often leads to end-stage renal disease (ESRD), high risk for cardiovascular disease, and high mortality. In the United States, the prevalence of CKD is estimated to be 11 percent.

Results from animal studies have suggested the potential reno-protective effects of active vitamin D and its analogs. Vitamin D is an important modulator of cellular proliferation, inflammation, differentiation, and immunity. Vitamin D reduces kidney injury by suppressing fibrosis, inflammation, and apoptosis, and by inhibiting multiple pathways known to play a role in kidney injury.

Dr. Pilz (Dr. Pilz! Again, not making this up!) estimated a significant 14 percent decrease in the relative risk of mortality per 10 nanograms per milliliter increase in D3 levels, indicating that higher vitamin D levels are associated with significantly improved survival in patients with chronic kidney disease. Further investigations are needed to uncover the potential life-saving mechanisms of vitamin D treatment for patients with CKD.

Lupus

Vitamin D3 inadequacy is prevalent in systemic lupus erythematosus (SLE), patients due to the avoidance of sunshine, photoprotection, renal insufficiency, and the use of medications, which alter the metabolism of vitamin D or down-regulate the functions of the vitamin D receptor.

Dr. Kamen and colleagues found significantly lower serum vitamin D3 levels among recently diagnosed Lupus patients compared to matched controls, and a high overall prevalence of vitamin D3 deficiency, even in the summer, likely, the study notes, due to the use of sunscreens, avoidance of sun exposure, darker skin pigment, and the limited amount of vitamin D obtained from dietary sources.

Vitamin D Deficiency and Lupus Incidence

Vitamin D regulates the immune system by being involved in interleukin-2 (IL-2) inhibition, antibody production, and lymphocyte proliferation. When administered in vivo, D3 is found to have a preventative effect on autoimmune diseases, such as murine lupus. Vitamin D deficiency is commonly reported in lupus.

As the immune-modulating effect of vitamin D is now established, it's logical to assume that vitamin D deficiency is a risk factor, rather than a consequence of lupus.

1,25-dihydroxy vitamin D can inhibit T cell proliferation and cytokine production, inhibit proliferation of activated B cells, and impair the generation of plasma cells. Differentiation of dendritic cells and production of type I interferon are important in the pathogenesis (manner of development) of lupus. Therefore, by positively affecting the immune system, vitamin D3 likely plays a preventive role in lupus.

Dr. Disanto and colleagues detected a clear seasonal distribution of beginnings for some immune-related diseases, including MS and lupus, in which a peak in April and a trough exactly 6 months later in October were found. These findings implicate a varying seasonal factor such as UVB radiation and subsequent vitamin D synthesis in disease etiology.

Vitamin D activity is dependent on the VDR (vitamin D receptor), a member of the nuclear hormone receptor superfamily. There are potential links between vitamin D deficiency and VDR polymorphisms that can affect VDR activity, having been evaluated as the probable cause of autoimmune diseases. The meta-analysis, conducted by Lee and colleagues addresses the link between VDR polymorphisms and rheumatoid arthritis and lupus susceptibility.

In comparison with many other cells and tissues that harbor VDR, muscles are some of the most sensitive tissues where vitamin D deficiency causes weakness and fatigue.

Vitamin D Insufficiency and Autoantibody Production in Lupus

The association between serum concentrations of vitamin D and the progression and development of autoimmune disorders has been focused on in numerous studies, revealing that disease activity and autoantibody production in lupus is aggravated by vitamin D insufficiency.

It can be reasonably concluded that vitamin D deficiency is a risk factor for the onset and development of disease activity in lupus. A study involving 378 patients with lupus from Europe to the Middle East conducted by Mok and colleagues showed an opposite relationship between 25-hydroxyvitamin D3 levels and disease activity scores.

In another report, Amital and colleagues revealed a significant inverse connection between the grade of lupus activity and serum vitamin D concentration—vitamin D deficiency contributed to the progression of active disease in patients with lupus.

In a study conducted on a large group of Australian patients, it was shown that vitamin D insufficiency was associated with higher disease activity, and a rise in serum vitamin D level was associated with reduced disease activity over time.

Vitamin D is a safe and inexpensive agent that is widely available. It could be beneficial as a disease suppressing intervention for lupus patients. Besides its potential benefit in improvement of SLE activity, vitamin D is known to present an immune-inflammatory-modulatory effect that can benefit musculoskeletal and cardiovascular manifestations of lupus.

Tabasi and colleagues isolated peripheral blood mononuclear cells (PBMCs) from 25 lupus patients and cultured them in 50 nanomoles of 1,25(OH)2 D3. The results showed that Vitamin D has regulatory effects on cell cycle progression, apoptosis (normal death of cells), and apoptosis-related molecules in lupus patients.

The results of the investigation conducted by Reynolds and colleagues demonstrate that vitamin D can positively modify endothelial function in lupus patients who are susceptible to cardiovascular diseases.

Abou-Raya and colleagues showed an inverse association between vitamin D levels and disease activity markers, with vitamin D levels lowest among patients with active lupus. They found an improvement in the levels of pro-inflammatory cytokines after 12 months of vitamin D supplementation compared to placebo.

Early vitamin D supplementation in animal SLE models presented immune regulating effects. For instance, dermatologic lesions, proteinuria, and anti-DNA were less in mice supplemented with vitamin D.

Macular Degeneration & Glaucoma

Dr. Kaufman of the Glaucoma Institute put D3 drops in the eyes of monkeys and reduced the intra-ocular pressures by 20-30 percent.

Experimental studies have suggested that vitamin D can control the expression of genes involved in oxidative stress, inflammation, and angiogenesis. In the macula, vitamin D may preserve the function of the retinal pigmentary epithelium and choroidal cells, through a paracrine/autocrine pathway. It is possible that the bioavailability of vitamin D circulating in blood is a limiting step in the protective effect of vitamin D.

On the other hand, observational studies, including population-based studies, suggest an association between vitamin D deficiency and a higher risk of both early or late macular degeneration. This is consistent for a role of vitamin D in the pathophysiology of macular degeneration. The apparent causal association between vitamin D and macular degeneration and glaucoma requires future clinical research.

Migraine Headache

There is ongoing research to prove that low vitamin D3 causes migraine. A recent report noted that 40 percent of sufferers with migraine have low vitamin D levels.

Another study, in the Journal of Headache Pain, discusses how migraines are more common at higher latitudes. This fact, and the pattern of migraine pain by season, suggests that migraines strike where sun exposure is decreased and vitamin D3 levels are reduced.

Scientists have now discovered that several brain areas—including the hypothalamus, which has been implicated in some types of headache—have receptors for D3, as well as enzymes that help convert it into the form your body uses, which explains why having inadequate D3 contributes to head pain.

Anecdotally, one researcher treated two women who had chronic migraines with vitamin D and calcium supplements, and their migraines went away.

"It is becoming more and more apparent to researchers that the vast majority of people are Vitamin D deficient—up to 70% or even 85% in some regions—and that symptoms of vitamin D deficiency are contributing to many of the chronic illnesses in western countries."
www.easy-immune-health.com/Vitamin-D-facts

Multiple Sclerosis

Multiple Sclerosis (MS) is climbing at an alarming rate in the northern latitudes while remaining almost unheard of near the equator.

Two large studies involving more than 187,000 women, which included 300 who developed MS during the study, evaluated the association between insufficient vitamin D3 and the risk of developing multiple sclerosis.

Women who had approximately 700 IU per day dietary vitamin D had a 33 percent lower incidence of multiple sclerosis when compared with those with lower vitamin D intake. Further, the women who took vitamin D3 supplements at a rate greater than 400 IU per day (specific details of quantity not provided) had a 41 percent reduced risk of developing MS compared to non-users.

Dr. Munger and colleagues evaluated serum vitamin D levels from blood samples of seven million U.S. military personnel and discovered that those with vitamin D levels greater than 100 nanomoles per liter had a 62 percent lower chance of developing MS.

The Finnish Maternity Cohort included more than 800,000 women and more than 1.5 million serum samples, serving as a basis for examining the association of vitamin D3 levels during pregnancy and MS risk. They mounted a study of 193 patients with a diagnosis of MS whose mothers had a serum sample from the pregnancy on record, and matched that population with 326 controls.

Vitamin D3 levels were low in both groups, but lower in the mothers of MS patients, and MS risk was shown to be 90 percent higher in the offspring of vitamin D deficient mothers, compared with offspring of mothers who were not vitamin D deficient, showing that insufficient vitamin D3 levels during pregnancy increases the risk of MS.

The association between neonatal vitamin D status and risk of MS was examined in a large study using data from the nationwide Danish MS Registry and the Danish Newborn Screening Biobank (DNSB). Data from 521 patients with MS and 972 controls were investigated. The analysis revealed that individuals with the highest risk of MS had less than 20.7 nanomoles per liter vitamin D3, and individuals with the lowest risk had more than 48.9 nanomoles per liter vitamin D3. Children born with vitamin D3 levels less than 30 nanomoles per liter are at especially high risk of developing MS.

Mokry and colleagues found that a genetically determined decrease in blood vitamin D level predicted increased MS susceptibility, while an increase of vitamin D levels by 50 percent decreased the odds of getting MS by approximately 50 percent. Similar findings were arrived at from a U.S. administrative claim database, and two population-based studies from Sweden.

Myasthenia Gravis

Myasthenia Gravis is a neuromuscular disorder that occurs when communication between nerve cells and muscles becomes impaired, causing weakness in the skeletal muscles, which are the muscles the body uses for movement.

A woman who had severe and refractory myasthenia gravis (MG), followed a mega-dose vitamin D treatment of 80,000 to 120,000 IU/day, and had her first complete remission after this treatment, while her vitamin D serum levels increased to 400-700 nanograms per milliliter!

This report reinforces the correlation between high-dose vitamin D and disease remission, and suggests the use of vitamin D as a safe and affordable treatment for autoimmune diseases.

Once again, what is needed is large, double-blind, placebo-controlled, randomized studies using high-dose vitamin D treatment for refractory autoimmune diseases.

Near- and Far-Sightedness

There are many anecdotal stories of people noting that their vision improved incidentally while taking high doses of D3 for another concern.

Obesity

An inadequate amount of D3 is an underpinning of obesity, which significantly contributes to other diseases, including Covid-19.

Obesity Pandemic

In 2010, complications related to obesity and excessive weight resulted in the death of at least 4 million people worldwide, and the decrease of the quality of life for 4 percent of the world's population every year.

According to the World Health Organization in 2014, 39 percent of the world's population was excessively overweight, and 13 percent were obese, with 43 million children under the age of 5, obese. The prevalence of vitamin D deficiency and insufficiency in overweight and obese patients ranges from 5.6 percent in Canada, to 96.0 percent in Germany.

Vitamin D deficiency is associated with an increased risk of diabetes, hypertension, heart failure, peripheral arterial disease, acute myocardial infarction, various forms of cancer, autoimmune and inflammatory diseases, decreased immune defenses, and increased mortality.

Vitamin D plays an essential role in the regulation of glucose homeostasis, insulin secretion mechanisms, and inflammation—all of which are compromised in obese people. The high rates of excessive body weight and obesity observed worldwide, coupled with vitamin D insufficiency, are closely interrelated problems indicating a pandemic.

Excessive body weight results in accumulation of adipose tissue, impaired adipocyte function, which leads to ectopic fat deposits in skeletal muscles, liver, and kidneys, dramatically increasing the risk of Type 2 Diabetes.

Add to that the development of adipocyte hypertrophy—the enlargement of adipose tissue to store excess energy intake including hyperplasia, cell number increase, and hypertrophy, cell size increase—and, further, an altered adipokine secretion profile (adipokines mediate inflammation and insulin resistance), and the world has a recipe for tragically bad health. It's an accident waiting to happen. And it has.

These changes result in the migration and transformation of macrophages developing adipose tissue inflammation—the synthesis of pro-inflammatory cytokines increases, and insulin resistance develops.

Vitamin D to the rescue (but you must promise to change dietary habits and get physical!). Vitamin D modulates the effect of the genes responsible for secretion of leptin and adiponectin. Further, vitamin D metabolites inhibit chronic immune-mediated inflammation by suppressing the production of the pro-inflammatory cytokines.

Long-term monitoring of obese patients receiving high-dose vitamin D supplements revealed an improvement of the adipose tissue inflammation.

Children and Obesity
Four countries are the leaders in the prevalence of childhood obesity: Greece, U.S., Italy, and Mexico. Most overweight and obese children and adolescents live in economically developed countries, particularly the U.S. The prevalence of obese or overweight American children and adolescents rose from approximately 6 percent in 1970 to currently greater than 18 percent.

But there is also a rise in obesity among children in countries with medium and low-income levels. The leading country is China, where 18 percent of the girls and 7 percent of the boys are obese. In Eastern European countries, the Russian Federation, and Turkey, the prevalence of excessive body weight and obesity is up to 19 percent among boys and up to 18 percent among girls.

Vitamin D Insufficiency Among Children and Adolescents
The prevalence of vitamin D insufficiency among children and adolescents with obesity is extremely high: 96.0 percent in Germany, 78.4 percent in the United States, and up to 92.0 percent in the Russian Federation.

Despite the overwhelming consensus that there's an urgent, life-sustaining, need to treat vitamin D insufficiency in obese patients, there is no common point of view on the dosage and duration of vitamin D supplementation.

> "Obesity appears to be a previously unrecognized risk factor for hospital admission and need for critical care."
> *Clinical Infectious Diseases*

Obesity Raises COVID-19 Risk

Researchers at New York University have observed that obesity is a risk factor for COVID-19 in patients under the age of 60.

Researchers looked at 3,615 patients admitted to their hospital from March 4 to April 4, 2020, and analyzed the body mass index (BMI) of the patients with confirmed COVID-19. A BMI of 18 to 25 is considered normal weight, 25 to 30 is overweight, and over 30 is obese.

What they discovered was that patients under 60 years of age with a BMI from 30 to 34 were two times more likely to be admitted to acute and critical care, compared with individuals with a BMI under 30. For patients in the same age-group with a BMI over 35, the risk was 3.6 times higher.

Nearly 40 percent of American adults under the age of 60 have a BMI of 30 or higher, making obesity a significant risk factor for COVID-19 hospitalizations.

Osteoporosis

Osteoporosis is a chronic, progressive disease of reduced bone mass and micro-architectural deterioration of bone, involving extensive fragility and an increase in fracture risk. Fracture risk is associated with increased bone remodeling, which results in bone resorption, loss of bone strength, and decrease of bone mineral density (BMD).

Osteoporosis patients who took 3,000 IU of vitamin D3 per day had their 25(OH)D increase and their parathyroid hormone (PTH) decrease more than those taking 800 IU per day. An increase of vitamin D3 greater than 75 nanomoles per liter resulted in normalized parathyroid hormone.

People over 60 years of age with vitamin D3 over 40 nanomoles per liter had better musculoskeletal function in the lower extremities than those with D3 less than 40 nanomoles per liter. There was, further, the beneficial effect of vitamin D supplementation resulting in fall prevention among older individuals with stable health by more than 20 percent!

Plantar Fasciitis

A man in Brazil had plantar fasciitis for two years. He started taking 25,000 IU D3 per day, and the plantar fasciitis went away in two weeks.

Pregnancy Complications

Pre-term births have gone up 36 percent in the last quarter of a century. This number has been reduced by half when pregnant women take 4,000 IU D3 per day.

An analysis of studies by the Medical University of South Carolina confirmed that a vitamin D level of at least 40 nanograms per milliliter may decrease pregnancy comorbidities.

Women with vitamin D levels of 40-60 nanograms per milliliter have a 46 percent lower preterm birth rate than the general population, with an even higher percentage among Hispanic and Black women. Also, the studies showed a 59 percent lower risk for premature birth by pregnant women with blood levels of vitamin D (25(OH)D) at or over 40 nanograms per milliliter by their third trimester than women who had levels below 20 nanograms per milliliter.

Other complications, such as pre-eclampsia, high blood pressure, and gestational diabetes have been reduced or eliminated by high intake of D3. Another area of major concern and need for research is the fact that strokes during and after pregnancy have risen 54 percent since 1994.

Schizophrenia

According to the National Institute of Mental Health, schizophrenia is one of the leading causes of disability worldwide. Symptoms include hallucinations, delusions, and cognitive problems.

Schizophrenic babies have low vitamin D3
Due to research that indicated there is more schizophrenia in areas with less sun, it was hypothesized that vitamin D deficiency is also a risk factor.

Research teams from Aarhus University in Denmark and the University of Queensland in Brisbane, Australia, found that newborn babies with vitamin D deficiency are at risk of developing schizophrenia later. An article in the journal, Scientific Reports, noted that vitamin D3 deficiency in newborn babies is likely responsible for eight percent of schizophrenia in Denmark.

According to the study, babies born with a vitamin D deficiency had a 44 percent higher risk of developing schizophrenia later in life. Since the fetus is totally reliant on the mother's vitamin D stores, these findings suggest that ensuring pregnant women have adequate levels of vitamin D will result in the prevention of a notable number of schizophrenia cases.

Scleroderma
Around 80 percent of scleroderma patients have a vitamin D3 deficiency. Taking a D3 supplement could help with many of the symptoms associated with the disease.

Sixty-five scleroderma patients underwent evaluation of vitamin D3 concentrations, none of whom were receiving vitamin D3 supplementation. Three of the 65 participants showed normal vitamin D3 values, with vitamin D3 insufficiency found in 43 cases, and deficiency in 19 cases.

The patients with vitamin D3 deficiency had lower diffusing lung capacity for carbon monoxide, higher pulmonary artery pressure, and longer disease duration, 13 years versus 9.4 years in comparison with patients with vitamin D3 insufficiency. None of the patients showed evidence of mal-absorption of vitamin D.

Seasonal Affective Disorder
Seasonal Affective Disorder is due to a lack of sunlight in the winter and thus, a lack of vitamin D3. As much as 100,000 IU of D3 per day in the "sunless" season has been recommended by health care professionals tracking this disorder, with the observation that high-dose vitamin D3 seems to be even more effective than light therapy.

Skin Disorders
Skin disorders such as dandruff, psoriasis, eczema, and fungus, are likely indications of inadequate D3. A doctor who had lifelong psoriasis started taking 50,000 IU D3 per day, and was cured of his disease in two months!

Strokes

Stroke is the world's second leading cause of death, with 6.7 million deaths annually. There's a 56 percent increased risk of stroke for people living in areas with weak sunlight.

Stroke is also the most frequent cause of permanent disability in adults, with half of all survivors discharged from the hospital into long-term or permanent care.

Currently, there is only one approved pharmacological agent available to treat stroke—recombinant tissue plasminogen activator (rtPA), which must be administered within a 4.5-hour window of stroke onset and only after a CT scan has diagnosed a thrombotic cause. Consequently, there is a desperate need to identify modifiable mechanisms capable of limiting the impact of acute stroke.

Targeting strokes inflammatory processes has been of intense interest to stroke researchers. However, one immune system modulating molecule that has received very little attention as a potential stroke therapy is vitamin D.

Studies have documented that patients with lower serum levels of vitamin D experience larger infarct volumes and worse functional outcomes following stroke (Tu, Wang, Turetsky, Daubail, and Park and all their colleagues), confirming that vitamin D plays a protective role during cerebral ischemia.

Following is a study of the effect of elevated baseline levels of vitamin D achieved by mega-doses of vitamin D given to vitamin D replete mice during the 5 days prior to induced stroke, in an analogous manner to high dose supplementation regimes in humans.

Male mice were randomly assigned to be administered either 1,25-VitD3 (100 nanograms per kg per day) or a placebo for 5 days prior to induced stroke. Stroke was induced via middle cerebral artery occlusion for 1 hour, followed by 23 hours re-perfusion. At 24 hours post-stroke, the infarct volume was assessed, functional deficit, expression of inflammatory mediators, and numbers of infiltrating immune cells. Supplementation with 1,25-VitD3 reduced infarct volume by 50 percent!

These data indicate that prior administration of exogenous vitamin D, even to vitamin D replete mice, can reduce infarct development and exert acute anti-inflammatory actions in the ischemic and re-perfused brain.

Tuberculosis
According to a study of 1,850 patients receiving antibiotic treatment led by Professor Adrian Martineau of Queen Mary University of London, Vitamin D3 has been shown to assist in clearing tuberculosis (TB) bacteria from the lungs of people who are multi-drug resistant (MDR TB).

Professor Martineau noted that multi-drug resistant TB is on the rise globally, notoriously difficult to treat, with a significantly worse prognosis than standard tuberculosis. This study offers the possibility that vitamin D3, which is safe and inexpensive, will benefit hard-to-treat patients by adding vitamin D3 to their antibiotic treatment. This boosts their immune system and helps the body clear the disease, rather than relying on antibiotics alone to kill the bacteria.

It's a superior approach when contrasted with the conventional tactic of trying to develop new antibiotics to keep ahead of the emerging drug-resistant bacteria, which is not very successful.

The World Health Organization estimates that ten million people developed tuberculosis in 2,017, and 1.6 million of them died. Existing antibiotic treatments are lengthy, costly, and often toxic, with serious side effects.

The researchers noted that the positive test results illustrate the potential for treatments that boost the immune system, and will improve outcomes in patients with drug-resistant bacterial infections.

Varicose Veins

Blood vessels help transport blood by alternately contracting and relaxing. Studies have shown that vitamin D plays a big role in helping promote relaxation of the vessels. It also keeps vessels supple, preventing them from becoming stiff. A lack of vitamin D, even in generally healthy people, is linked to stiffer arteries and an inability of blood vessels to relax.

These facts add to the body of evidence that lack of vitamin D leads to compromised vascular health, contributing to high blood pressure and the risk of cardiovascular disease. Study participants who increased their vitamin D levels improved their vascular health and lowered their blood pressure.

There are many anecdotal reports of varicose veins shrinking and even disappearing on high doses of D3, even when people have been taking high-dose vitamin D3 for another reason.

Vertigo

A study published in 2015 found treating vitamin D deficiency helped reduce the recurrence of benign paroxysmal positional vertigo (BPPV).

BPPV is a balance disorder that occurs when calcium crystals become dislodged from their location in the inner ear, resulting in sudden bouts of dizziness, a spinning sensation, lightheadedness, and nausea.

Scientists confirmed that vitamin D3 receptors are to be found on calcium channel transport systems in the inner ear and they help regulate proper calcium balance. This contributes to explaining the role of vitamin D3 in maintaining proper ear function.

Regarding the 93 participants in the study, the researchers concluded: "Improvement of serum 25-hydroxyvitamin D3 levels is associated with substantial decrease in recurrence of BPPV (vertigo)."

Vitiligo

Vitiligo is when the immune system attacks and destroys the melanocytes in the skin, removing the skin's color pigment.

A small study of 16 people with pronounced vitiligo had a very low mean of D3 at 18.4 nanograms per milliliter at the outset of the treatment. After 6 months of 35,000 IU vitamin D3 per day, their D3 levels increased significantly to a mean of 132.5 nanograms per milliliter.

The results of repigmentation were dramatic for most of the participants. Although two patients showed no repigmentation, four patients showed nearly 25 percent repigmentation, five patients showed 26–50 percent repigmentation, five patients showed 51–75 percent repigmentation, while none showed more than 75 percent repigmentation.

As was noted in the study, "Enhancing both innate and adaptive immunity is a significant advantage of high-dose vitamin D3 therapy for autoimmune disorders over the current treatment with immunosuppressive drugs."

This study makes it apparent that, at least for patients with autoimmune disorders like vitiligo and psoriasis, a daily dose of 35,000 IU of vitamin D is a safe and effective therapeutic approach for reducing disease activity.

Wounds

Vitamin D3 is absolutely essential for wounds to heal. If you sustain an injury, the skin's cells require higher amounts of vitamin D, which has several roles in the process of healing.

Vitamin D controls the genes that promote the creation of cathelicidin, the antimicrobial peptide the immune system uses to fight off infections. Vitamin D deficiency compromises immune function, providing an inlet for harmful bacteria, while, at the same time, wounds tend to cause a deficiency in vitamin D.

A study conducted by researchers at the Evangelical University Hospital of Curitiba in Brazil looked into the relationship between vitamin D insufficiency and healing with a group of 26 patients who had leg ulcers, and a control group of the same size.

Half of the ulcer group received vitamin D for a period of two months, while the other half was given a placebo.

All the participants in the study who had wounds had a vitamin D deficiency, while the members of the control group did not. The participants who received the vitamin D supplementation saw a decrease in the size of the ulcer, the participants who took a placebo had no significant change.

The researchers concluded that patients with ulcers are more likely to have a vitamin D deficiency. There exists a trend toward better healing in people who undergo a vitamin D regimen to counter their deficiencies.

*   *   *

Whew! In other words, we need our D3!

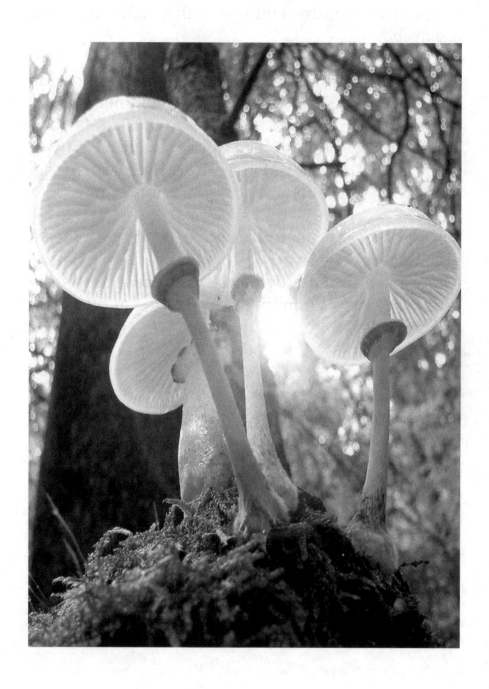

Chapter Three

D3's Perfect Companion—K2

A Danish scientist by the name of Henrik Dam discovered vitamin K eighty-four years ago while investigating the effects on chickens of a low-fat diet. The bleeding tendencies in the chickens on the low-fat diet were prevented when they were fed a diet with normal levels of fat, with vitamin K added. Thus, vitamin K became vitamin K for the German word koagulation. It was then discovered that vitamin K had two forms: phylloquinone, named vitamin K_1, and menaquinone, named vitamin K_2.

A half-cup serving of broccoli contains the daily recommended minimum amount of vitamin K (150 mcg), whereas spinach and kale contain 3.5 to 5 times as much. To check if you have sufficient vitamin K, you can ask your physician to check your prothrombin time (how long it takes blood to clot).

Show Me the K1:

Foods high in K_1 include:

Kale (cooked) – 443% daily value per serving

Mustard Greens (cooked) – 346% daily value per serving

Swiss Chard (raw) – 332% daily value per serving

Collard Greens (cooked) – 322% daily value per serving

Spinach (raw) – 121% daily value per serving

Broccoli (cooked) – 92% daily value per serving

Vitamin K_2 comes from bacteria. Fermented foods are the best source of vitamin K_2. Amounts of K_2 for fermented foods vary widely, depending on the fermenting process, but natto is the leader in K_2 availability. It's generally about 10 mg (that's milligrams, not micrograms!) of K_2 per 100 grams of natto.

A few other fermented foods among a host of hundreds are:

sauerkraut

kombucha

aqua kefir

dairy kefir

fermented pickles

dosa

kimchi

miso

soy sauce

Tabasco sauce

tempeh

vinegar
Worcestershire sauce
And the list goes on....

Both K_1 and K_2 are essential to maintain blood hemostasis and optimal bone and heart health, as they induce calcium use by proteins. Vitamin K_2 is essential for calcium use, helping build strong bones and inhibiting arterial calcification.

Vitamin K is essential for the functioning of eight proteins involved in blood clotting. It's required for coagulation and anticoagulation factors and for binding osteocalcin (a protein) to hydroxyapatite (the chief structural element of vertebrate bone). Vitamin K is considered to be required for the function of the protein, matrix Gla protein (MGP), which is an inhibitor of vascular mineralization, and has a role in bone organization.

Vitamin K is a family of structurally related molecules derived from different sources, that share the same nucleus—methylated naphthoquinone (menadione). The different molecules have side chains of different composition and length, with varying potencies and absorption efficiencies.

A study by Kaneki and colleagues proved that increased consumption of vitamin K_2 in the form of MK-7 led to more activated osteocalcin, linked to increased bone-matrix formation and bone mineral density, resulting in lower risk of hip fracture. In a 3-year study of 944 women, 20 to 79 years old, it was demonstrated that MK-7-rich natto was associated with the preservation of bone mineral density.

Inadequate calcium intake leads to decreased bone mineral density, which can increase the risk of bone fractures. Supplemental calcium promotes bone mineral density and strength and can prevent osteoporosis (ie, porous bones), particularly in older adults and postmenopausal women. However, elevated consumption of calcium supplements raises the risk for heart disease and has been connected to accelerated deposits of calcium in blood vessel walls and soft tissues.

Enter, K2! It has been shown to inhibit arterial calcification and arterial stiffening. Increasing vitamin K2 intake is a probable means of lowering calcium-associated health risks.

This is problematic though, since the 1950s the consumption of vitamin K has decreased. Even a diet as well-balanced as one can get still may not provide enough. This is due to modern manufacturing processes, wherein the supply of K2 has significantly dropped, making supplements a reliable way to be assured of adequate intake.

A clinical study with vitamin K2 supplementation showed an improvement in arterial elasticity and regression in age-related arterial stiffening. Through the activation of K–dependent proteins, vitamin K2 can optimize calcium use in the body, preventing negative health issues associated with increased calcium intake.

Vitamin K2: Essential Role

Bone is composed of a hard outer shell and a spongy matrix of inner tissues. Your entire skeleton is replaced every 7 to 10 years. This process of rebuilding your bones in an ongoing process is referred to as "remodeling." During this remodeling, your body releases calcium from the bone into the bloodstream to meet your body's metabolic needs, allowing the bone to perform the virtually mystical process of altering the size and shape of your bones as they grow, or as they repair from injuries.

This remodeling is regulated by osteoblasts—cells that build up the skeleton, and osteoclasts—cells that break down the skeleton. As long as the bone-forming activity, referred to as absorption, is greater than the breakdown of bone, referred to as resorption, the process of maintaining a healthy bone structure is maintained.

Osteoblasts produce osteocalcin. Osteocalcin takes calcium from your blood as it circulates, and binds it to the bone matrix, making the skeleton stronger and less susceptible to fracture. But the newly made osteocalcin is inactive—vitamin K2 activates it so it can bind calcium.

The other vitally important action of vitamin K2 is that it keeps calcium from accumulating in the walls of blood vessels. Because calcification occurs in the vessel walls, it leads to thickening of the wall via calcified plaques, and to the typical progression of atherosclerosis, which, of course, is associated with a higher risk of cardiovascular events.

The vitamin K-dependent protein, matrix GLA protein (MGP), is a calcification inhibitor, produced by the cells of vascular smooth muscles, regulating the potentially fatal accumulation of calcium.

With this "supervisory" role of K2, keeping calcium out of the walls of blood vessels, the calcium is then is available for multiple other roles in the body, leaving the arteries healthy and flexible.

A study in Rotterdam of 4,807 healthy men and women over 55 years of age, evaluated the relationship between dietary intake of vitamin K and aortic calcification, heart disease, and all-cause mortality. At least 32 micrograms per day of vitamin K2 was associated with a 50 percent reduction in death from cardiovascular issues related to arterial calcification, and a 25 percent reduction in all-cause mortality.

In another study of 16,000 healthy women, 49 to 70 years of age, the data showed that eight years of a high intake of natural vitamin K2 reduced cardiovascular events. For every 10 mcg of dietary vitamin K2 in the forms of menaquinone 7 (MK-7), menaquinone 8 (MK-8), and menaquinone 9 (MK-9), the risk of coronary heart disease was reduced by 9 percent.

A double-blind, randomized clinical trial investigating the effects of supplemental MK-7 in a three-year period of a group of 244 postmenopausal Dutch women found that a daily dose of 180 mcg was enough to improve bone mineral density, bone strength, and cardiovascular health. Achieving this clinically relevant improvement required a minimum of two years of supplementation.

Vitamin K_1 Compared to K_2

Although vitamin K_1 can activate MGP, it is much less efficient because it is transported to the liver first to activate coagulation proteins. To render the proteins regulating calcium active, a sufficient amount of vitamin K_2 is necessary.

If at least 32 mcg of vitamin K_2 is present in the diet, then the risks for blood-vessel calcification and heart problems are significantly lowered, and the elasticity of the vessel wall is increased. Moreover, beneficial effects of vitamins D and K on the elastic properties of the vessel wall in postmenopausal women have been seen in clinical trials.

In general, the typical Western diet contains insufficient amounts of vitamin K_2 to activate MGP adequately, which means that approximately 30 percent of the proteins that can be activated by vitamin K_2 remain inactive. The percentage of K deficiency increases with age.

Although vitamin K_1 is present in green leafy vegetables, only 10 percent of the total amount is absorbed from that source in the diets of people in industrialized countries. The only exception seems to be the Japanese diet, particularly for the portion of the population consuming high quantities of foods rich in vitamin K_2, such as natto.

Suboptimal levels of vitamin K_2 disadvantage the activation of specific proteins that are dependent on vitamin K_2. If those proteins cannot perform their function in keeping calcium in the bones and preventing calcium deposits in soft tissues, that is to say, the arterial walls during situations of increased calcium intake, then general health, and, in particular, cardiovascular health, may suffer due to an inefficient and misdirected use of calcium in the body.

That issue is remedied with the right amount of vitamin K_2 added to a high-calcium regimen. Vitamin K_2 promotes arterial flexibility by preventing accumulation of arterial calcium, and supplementation with it could correct calcium amounts in the body that are out of balance.

D_3 promotes the production of vitamin K-dependent proteins, so vitamin K_2 can ensure that calcium is absorbed easily and reaches the bone mass, and prevent arterial calcification, keeping your heart and bones healthy. K_2 regulates normal blood clotting, while D_3 supports a healthy immune system, and supports muscle function.

Ratio of Vitamin K to Vitamin D

It's generally recommended to have nearly the same amount of vitamin K as vitamin D. If the vitamin K is measured in micrograms (mcg) and the vitamin D is measured in IU, take 100 mcg vitamin K for each 4,000 IU of D.

> "The pituitary, pineal, and hypothalamus glands are behind the eyes, where they can be exposed to direct sunlight. When UV light strikes these glands, they cause the body to produce a host of hormones; calcitonin, serotonin, and melatonin, and enzymes such as inositol triphosphate, that are crucial for life."
> *Robert Barefoot*

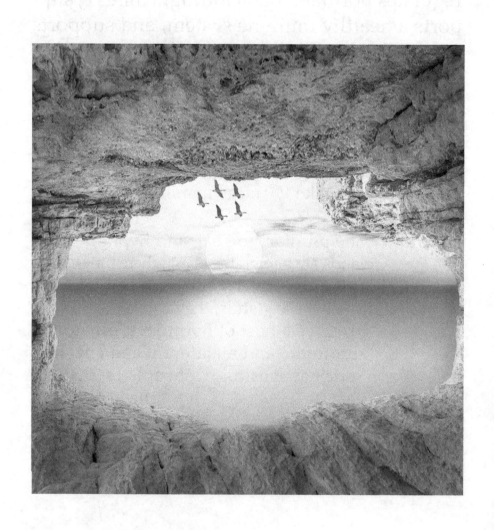

Chapter Four

Magnesium —
A Significant Component
Of Your Health

We now come to the extremely relevant contribution of magnesium to your health, especially in conjunction with D3 and K2.

Why is it so important? Because D3 cannot metabolize without adequate magnesium. The D3 simply remains stored and inactive in your body. As much as 50 percent of Americans are magnesium deficient. Keep in mind that magnesium is the fourth most abundant mineral in the human body after calcium, potassium, and sodium, and it must be adequate.

Deficiency in either magnesium or D3 is associated with numerous health issues, including skeletal deformities, cardiovascular diseases, and metabolic syndrome.

The recommended daily allowance for magnesium is 420 mg for men and 320 mg for women. But the standard diet in the United States contains only about 50 percent of that amount. Why? Because the availability of magnesium in natural foods has decreased over the last few decades due to industrialized farming, and because of changes in dietary habits that include processed foods and junk (non)food.

A professor of medicine at Vanderbilt University Medical Center, Dr. Qi Dai, reported on the relationship between magnesium intake and vitamin D levels in over 12,000 individuals taking part in the National Health and Nutrition Examination Survey (NHANES) 2001 to 2006 study.

His study revealed that individuals with high levels of magnesium, whether from dietary sources or supplements, were less likely to have low levels of vitamin D. He also found an association between adequate magnesium intake and a reduction in cardiovascular disease and, further, an association between magnesium and a reduction in bowel cancer.

Show Me the Magnesium
Foods high in magnesium include:
almonds
bananas
beans
broccoli
brown rice

cashews
flaxseed
green vegetables
mushrooms
cashews
Brazil nuts
peanuts
oatmeal
pumpkin seeds
sesame seeds
soybeans
sunflower seeds
sweet corn
tofu
whole grains

"A few grams of magnesium chloride
every few hours will clear nearly all
acute illnesses. I have seen flu cases
healed in 24-48 hours with 3 grams
of magnesium chloride taken
every 6-8 hours."

Dr. Mark Sircus

Clues that You May Have
A Magnesium Deficiency

A variety of painful conditions may be indicators of a
magnesium deficiency, especially if these conditions
present as tense and/or tight, including muscle cramps,
chronic back pain, migraines, tendonitis, and fibromyalgia, to name a few.

Not only physical manifestations, but also tense emotions such as anger, aggression, ADHD, insomnia, and obsessive-compulsive disorder can be signs of magnesium deficiency.

"Patients with diagnoses of depression, epilepsy, diabetes mellitus, tremor, Parkinsonism, arrhythmias, circulatory disturbances (stroke, cardiac infarction, arteriosclerosis), hypertension, migraine, cluster headache, cramps, neuro-vegetative disorders, abdominal pain, osteoporosis, asthma, stress-dependent disorders, tinnitus, ataxia, confusion, chronic fatigue syndrome, kidney stones, preeclampsia, or weakness, might also be consequences of the magnesium deficiency syndrome."

Kerri Knox, RN

Many people with the foregoing disorders and diseases had signs of magnesium deficiency long before the disease became defined.

But a major complication is that few medical professionals are knowledgeable about magnesium deficiency and have sometimes made it worse. They know about the recent hue and cry regarding vitamin D3, and so they tell their patients to supplement with vitamin D. Then the problems potentially get worse when the individual does not also supplement with the necessary, balancing, magnesium (or K2).

"I recommend magnesium bicarbonate,
which is a liquid form of magnesium.
Magnesium bicarbonate is the ultimate
mitochondrial cocktail."
Dr. Mark Sircus

Your Magnesium Supplementation

As noted, the minimum required amount of magnesium for men is 420 mg. per day, and for women, 320 mg. per day. If you're intending to increase your magnesium intake, please plan on doing so gradually, or you will quickly discover the "clearing factor" of diarrhea if magnesium intake is increased too much, too fast.

"Magnesium deficiency shuts down vitamin D
synthesis and metabolism pathways."
Dr. Qi Dai

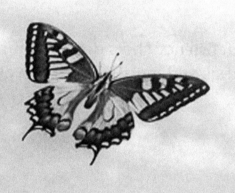

Chapter Five

Bring Home the Boron

*A*nd rounding out the perfect immune support recipe, let's not leave out boron!

Findings suggest that boron acts on at least three separate metabolic sites because it compensates for perturbations induced by vitamin D3 deficiency, augments major mineral content in bone, and, independently of vitamin D3, enhances some aspects of cartilage maturation.

Boron is used for building strong bones, treating osteoarthritis, as an aid for building muscles and increasing testosterone levels, and for improving thinking skills and muscle coordination. Boron helps increase serum vitamin D levels.

Boron seems to affect the way the body handles other minerals such as calcium, magnesium, and phosphorus. It also appears to increase estrogen levels in postmenopausal women and healthy men. Estrogen is thought to be helpful in maintaining healthy bones and mental function. Boric acid, a common form of boron, can kill yeast that causes vaginal infections. And boron is believed to have antioxidant effects.

Here's a short list of the health risks associated with boron deficiency:

Ankylosing spondylitis, arthritis, low bone density, abnormal bone development, increased urinary calcium excretion, embryonic development problems, low immune function, osteoporosis, rheumatoid arthritis, tooth decay, impaired wound healing.

Boron helps your body absorb magnesium, while boron deficiency symptoms overlap with D3 deficiency symptoms.

Boron increases the useful life of vitamin D3.

One study found that a solution of 3 percent boric acid applied to deep wounds reduced healing time by 70 percent.

Boron keeps teeth and gums healthy, stimulating bone and tissue repair and reducing inflammation.

A boron paste applied to diabetic foot ulcers accelerated their healing.

Boron, independently of vitamin D3, enhances cartilage remodeling.

Arthritic bones contain less boron than healthy bones.

Boron reduces the cytokines involved in causing lung and breast cancers, insulin resistance, coronary disease, obesity, and depression.

Boron is helpful in preventing prostate cancer, suppressing the levels of PSA.

Boron deficiency in animals and humans negatively affects brain activity with attention span, short-term memory, and coordination.

Boron and 10mg per day of vitamin B6 increased kidney stone elimination and decreased pain.

Boron supplements increased the mineral density of athletes' bones.

Boric acid helps arthritic dogs be in less pain and move better.

France has a very high average daily boron intake at 10 milligrams per day. The average intake in the UK is .8 to 5 milligrams per day. France has half the rate of rheumatoid arthritis and ankylosing spondylitis as the UK.

U.S. average intake is 1.5 milligrams per day. Be sure to take your boron supplement!

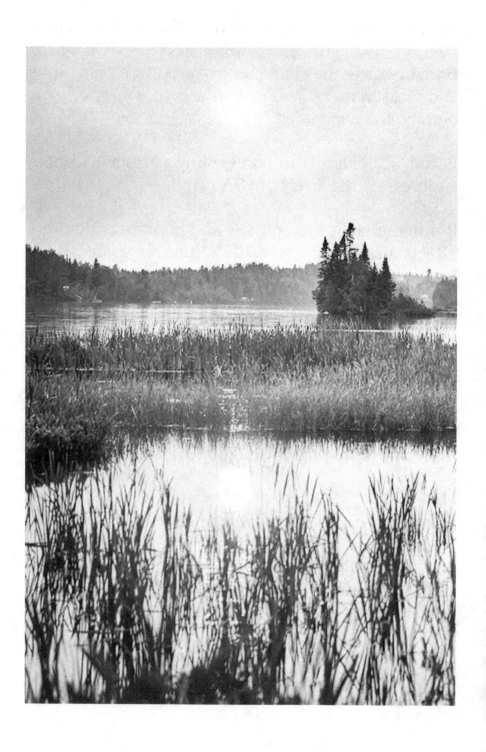

Chapter Six

And a Pinch of Zinc

*I*t's estimated that half the world's farming land is zinc deficient, and thus, half the world's population—or more—is zinc deficient.

Crops are grown in zinc-deficient soil, although zinc fertilization increases crop yields while providing enough zinc in crops for people to not be deficient.

There are over 300 zinc-containing enzymes. Zinc is a cofactor that helps vitamin D3 function. The recommended daily allowance of zinc is 10 mg, with the suggested upper level noted as 40 mg per day. Beans and nuts are excellent sources of zinc.

The thymus uses a considerable amount of zinc, and it's believed that zinc deficiency is the leading cause of infant mortality, due to malfunctioning immune systems because of the malfunctioning, zinc deficient, thymus.

Zinc lozenges reduce the length of a cold by 50 percent.

As we age, the thymus shrinks. However, in a study with mice that were given zinc and melatonin, their thymuses began to grow....

That's amazing!

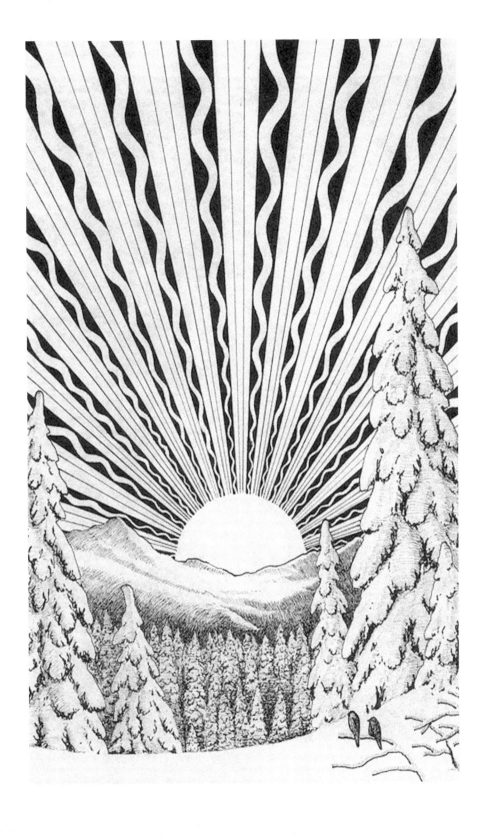

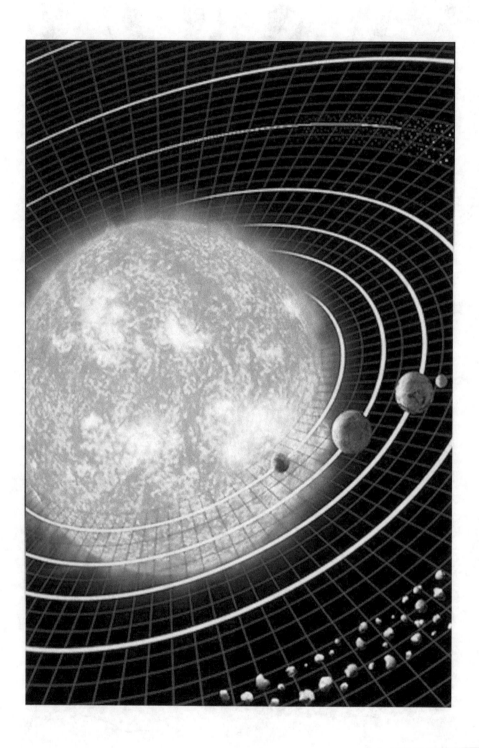

Chapter Seven

The Burning Question

*I*s not the burning question, "Why are we deficient in D3?"

Jeff T. Bowles, author of *The Miraculous Cure for and Prevention of All Diseases*, and several other books, presented some interesting history, a thumbnail sketch I note here.

In the 1920s, the "vitamin craze" started, following Casimir Funk's discovery and development of a vitamin D and A supplement, as mentioned before, called, "Oscodal."

At the same time, hospitals, which had previously played a charitable role in society, began to shift the charitable role to one of prestigious facilities, expensive centers of health, science, and technology, attractive to the upper-middle class who could afford to, and who were willing to, spend money for their health care.

Between 1909 and 1932, the number of hospital beds increased six times as fast as the population. At the same time, the average person was taking 25 mg (1,000,000 IU!) of vitamin D2 or D3 per day—without vitamin D toxicity. But, even more to the point, without getting sick with the previously prevalent diseases.

Everything from hot dogs to bread to milk to beer was being fortified with vitamin D.

Because everyone was healthy and happy—it was, after all, the roaring 20s—hospitals lay fallow, emptying, and causing the medical authorities enough stress to give them ulcers. So, what did they do? They mounted the propaganda that vitamin D "may be toxic." They then figured out a clever way to manipulate the public by changing the unit of measure for crucial, health-providing, vitamins: D, E, and A.

Before this nefarious move, all supplements were measured in micrograms and milligrams, which they changed to "International Units" or "IU."As I noted above, people were suddenly taking one-million IUs of D3, and it indeed did sound like it would likely be toxic. (500 MG of vitamin C would math out to 20,000,000 vitamin D IUs. Why didn't people think about that?)

Because the populace had been in the habit of trusting their medical professionals, and even the doctors themselves believed the authorities to whom they answered, this ploy was—and is—wildly successful.

Hospital beds were soon full again, with millions upon millions of people, since then until now, deathly ill and dying for lack of simple, essential nutrients, with a cost to society of untold trillions of dollars. And, more to the point, untold pain and anguish.

This is the world we're living in today, with hospitals everywhere over-full and the human family suffering in the throes of an (avoidable) pandemic.

"Despite being admonished by the courts and Congress, government agencies still refuse to abide by the law. They want control of the sale of vitamins for the benefit of the drug industry, which they want to package as drugs. News stories have demonstrated how important vitamins have been to society since their discovery, and how much money has been spent trying to promote, patent, exploit and suppress these vitamins."

Robert Barefoot
Disease Conspiracy

In the 1980s, the skin cancer scare took over, and people began to stay out of the sun. If they went into the sun, they slathered themselves with sunscreen. The result of this, several years down the road is, again, that inadequate sun causes disease. And even worse, as it has now been unambiguously shown that sunscreen causes skin cancer.

Stranger than Fiction

But here is an interesting twist to the story ... the FDA recently mandated a change of IU back to microgram and milligram (mcg/mg)! You ought to be seeing your supplements of D, E, and A, in nice, tidy, measurements, the same across the board with your other supplements.

I quote:

"In the new regulation for the nutrition facts label, FDA has replaced the unit 'IU' for vitamin A, vitamin D, and vitamin E with the metric unit. The unit for vitamin A is changed to micrograms of retinol activity equivalents (mcg RAE), vitamin E is milligram of alpha-tocopherol (mg), while Vitamin D is now changed to microgram. This regulation came into effect on Jan. 1, 2020, for companies with U.S. $10 million or more in annual sales, and Jan 1, 2021, for companies with less than $10 million in annual sales."

* * *

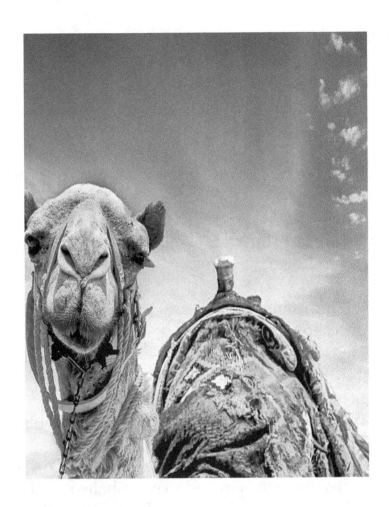

Saving the Earth

If you've noticed that in this book there are no references to animal products. Folows are a few zoonotic reasons why ("*75 percent of all emerging infectious diseases are zoonotic,*" www.livescience.com, due to human exploitation of wild and domestic animals):

Spanish Flu – Avian

HIV/AIDS – Chimpanzee

SARS – Bats/civet cats

MERS – Camels, bats

Swine Flu – Pigs

Avian Influenza – Birds–more than a dozen forms of bird flu

Other forms of Influenza – Horses, pigs, wild aquatic animals, minks

Ebola – Chimpanzees, gorillas, fruit bats, monkeys, forest antelope, porcupines

Creutzfeldt-Jakob Disease – Cattle

Anthrax – Cattle, sheep, goats, camels, horses, pigs

Bovine Spongiform Encephalopathy/Mad Cow Disease – Herbivore cows forced to cannibalism, fed their dead peers, roadkill, and other dead and rotten animals

Covid-19 – bats/pangolins

I'm sure you're able to connect the dots without my going on and on.

A Few of Your Author's Miscellaneous Thoughts

I suspect that Covid-19 "hovers"—that it stays where it's been put for a surprisingly long time. For this reason, I feel that the lines at the likes of Costco and Trader Joe's are verrrry unwise places to hang out. I've not been to Trader Joe's for two months, a record, since I fell in love with it three years ago. (I'll be glad to go back, whenever that may be.)

As mentioned, but let me make a point of it again, soils are depleted. This is why nutrition is suffering, and you need to thoughtfully supplement.

Another point is the question of UV lamps, which do, indeed, make the body produce D3. But there is controversy over their safety, so do your research before you go this route.

It's a great pity that Covid-19 patients are, of necessity, indoors, and not getting any sun. If there's any possibility to get them in the sun, even a few minutes a day, it could be remarkably beneficial (and the same for the health care providers that are out in the sun with the patients).

The sun's UV rays that produce vitamin D are blocked by glass. Yes, even clear glass. Move outside and get your rays. Of course you have to take off your glasses, why do you even ask?

Vitamin D3 is safe and affordable—undoubtedly the most inexpensive life insurance you can invest in.

* * *

A few of you may be curious about my own intake and experience of these nutrients:

I'm taking high-dose Vitamin D3 and K2. My D3 is made from lichen. Yes, this is a plant-based D3, for anyone who wants to insist there's no plant-based D3. The K2 is made from natto. I'm taking 6,000 IU (150 mcg) morning and evening of D3 and 150 mcg of K2 (= 6,000 IU), morning and evening.

I take the same amount of both nutrients to support their symbiotic relationship. I've seen supplements with both nutrients together. Some of these supplements are close to this ratio, and some are not, so it requires a bit of attention.

I'm not going to suggest what quantity you need to take. You've read this book, and you must come to your own conclusions about what seems right, or work it out with your naturopathic healthcare provider.

Magnesium: Calm brand, 2 teaspoons – 325 mg. in water in the evening. I also take a nightly bath with Epsom salts.

Epsom Salt, named for a bitter saline spring at Epsom in Surrey, England, is pure mineral magnesium sulfate.

And I have a spray magnesium which I spritz on forearms and feet/shins on occasion. It says right on the bottle it's not oily, but I'd like to see, then, what they consider oily.

Boron: 6 mg. liquid
Zinc: 50 mg.

I started taking the high-dose D3-K2 for preventative measures, to shore up my immune system. I've been taking the 12,000 IUs per day for about 6 weeks as I write this, and I have these further fun facts to share. I absolutely stopped have middle-of-the-night leg cramps—even if I've been on a ladder for hours during the day, which I often am this time of year.

I've had a little plantar wart (I guess it is) on the bottom of my left baby toe for about five months, which has been most irritatingly painful. It now has been simply shrinking away. That's very nice.

And my eyes! I have glasses for near and glasses for far. Lately, I sometimes will be working away for hours at my writing (as always), and then, intending to make a cup of tea, I look for my "see far" glasses, only to discover I've been wearing them! Which means my seeing near is improving, but erratically. And then, sometimes when I'm outside, wearing my "seeing far" glasses, things are blurry. I take the glasses off, and everything becomes more clear. Super interesting!

Hot & Humid

This last winter, I had a persistent cough. I didn't feel sick, I just had a cough, a big part of why I started taking high-dose D3-K2.

A friend of mine also had a nagging cough. He emailed me saying he'd read that this was the driest year on record for the state of Washington. He turned on his humidifier, and his cough went away overnight. I plugged in my little Vicks humidifier, and indeed, my nagging cough disappeared in a couple of days. After six weeks of irritation.

One cannot help but suspect that this dryness accelerated Washington state's Covid-19 outbreak. I hear from other sources that Covid-19 thrives in dry cold. So! Spend some time in the sun, and stay humid, dear reader.

And You?

I would like to hear about your experiences if you decide to engage in anything I've presented in these pages.

I only have one heart's desire, and that is that anyone who reads this feels inspired and empowered, while living a life filled with health, happiness, and kindness.

My Gift for You ....

As a thank you for reading *Save Your Life with the the Dynamic Duo – D3 and K2*, I have a gift for you, *Save Your Life with Stupendous Spices*. To receive your ebook, type in the following link:

www.BlytheAyne.com/StupendousSpices

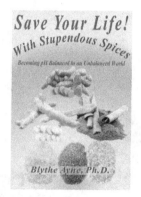

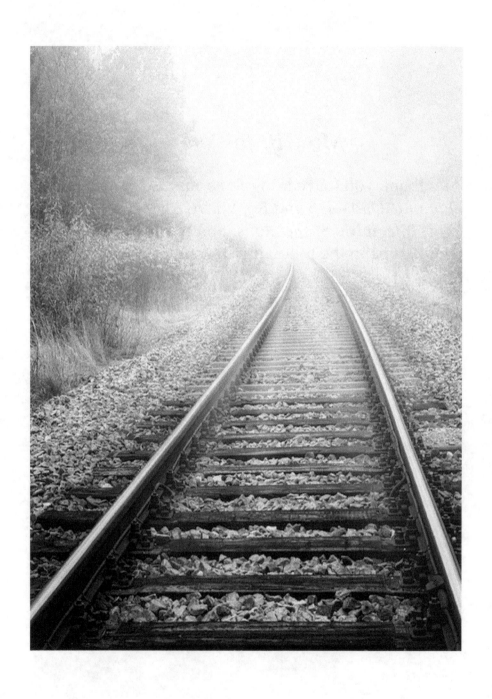

Glossary:

25-hydroxyvitamin D (25(OH)D) – Vitamin D3.

Adipocyte Hypertrophy – Adipocyte cells are the cells that compose adipose tissue, that stores energy as fat. Hypertrophy describes one of the ways cells adapt to environmental changes.

Aldosterone – a corticosteroid hormone (hormones produced in the adrenal cortex) which stimulates absorption of sodium by the kidneys, regulating water and salt balance.

Angiotensin – a protein that promotes aldosterone secretion, which tends to raise blood pressure.

Apoptosis – normal death of cells.

Autocrine – cell acting on the surface of itself.

Cathelicidins – small, cationic, positively charged ions, that are antimicrobial peptides (compounds consisting of two or more amino acids linked in a chain), found in humans and other species. These proteolytically (proteins broken down into simpler compounds) activated peptides are part of the innate (immediate) immune system of many vertebrates. Cathelicidins serve a critical role in immune defense against invasive bacterial infection. The cathelicidin family of antimicrobial peptides (AMPs) also includes the defensins.

Defensins – small cysteine-rich cationic proteins across cellular life, including vertebrate and invertebrate animals, plants, and fungi. They are host defense peptides, displaying direct antimicrobial activity or immune signaling activities, or both.

Diastolic Blood Pressure – is the pressure of the blood in the arteries when the heart is filling. It is the lower of two blood pressure measurements

Endocrine – cells that release hormones that act on distant target cells.

Endoplasmic Reticulum Stress – The endoplasmic reticulum is an ultramicroscopic organelle of plant and animal cells consisting of a system of membrane-bound cavities in the cytoplasm. Endoplasmic reticulum stress (ERS), generally due to excess weight and obesity, contributes to the development of insulin resistance, and other health complications.

Endothelium – Along with acting as a semi-permeable membrane, the endothelium maintains vascular tone and regulates oxidative stress by releasing mediators, such as nitric oxide, endothelin, and prostacyclin. It also controls local angiotensin-II activity.

Hydroxyapatite – Chief mineral component of bones and teeth, providing their strength and rigidity.

Interleukin-2 (IL-2) – a cytokine-signaling molecule in the immune system. It regulates the activities of white blood cells (leukocytes, lymphocytes) responsible for immunity. IL-2 is part of the body's natural response to microbial infection, discriminating between "foreign" and "self."

Inverse Correlation – The more of A the less of B, the less of A, the more of B.

Lymphocyte – A type of white blood cell or leukocyte that is divided into three types:
• B-lymphocytes, producing antibodies in the humoral immune response
• T-lymphocytes, participating in the cell-mediated immune response
• The null group, containing natural killer cytotoxic cells that participate in the innate immune response.

Macrophage – a large white blood cell that is an important part of our immune system that 'eats' bacteria, viruses, fungi, and parasites. They are born from white blood cells called monocytes, produced by stem cells in our bone marrow.

Matrix Gla Protein (MGP) – K_2 dependent, GLA (gamma linolenic acid)-containing proteins. Binds to calcium ions, acts as an inhibitor of vascular mineralization, and plays a role in bone organization.

Metabolite – a small molecule involved in metabolism.
Mole – the amount of a substance that contains the same number of particles (molecules or ions) that is in 12 grams of carbon. One mole always contains the same number of particles.

Nanomole – 1billionth of a mole.

Nanogram – one billionth (1/1,000,000,000) of a gram.

Nitric Oxide Synthesis – Nitric oxide is synthesized from the amino acid L-arginine by the enzyme nitric oxide synthase. The main site of the molecule's synthesis is the endothelium, which is the inner layer of blood vessels. The molecule is also produced by other types of cells.

Osteocalcin – Calcium-binding substance, produced by osteoblasts—essential to bone mineralization and used to identify osteoporosis. May act as a hormone to increase insulin production and insulin sensitivity.

Oxidative Stress – An imbalance between free radicals—oxygen-containing molecules with an uneven number of electrons—and the antioxidants in your body.

Pathogenesis – the manner of development.

Pathophysiology – the disordered physiological processes associated with disease or injury.

Parathyroid Hormone (PTH) – A polypeptide hormone secreted by the parathyroid glands, influencing calcium and phosphorus metabolism and bone formation.

Paracrine – cells that act on nearby cells.

Proinflammatory Cytokines – produced predominantly by activated macrophages, involved in the up-regulation of inflammatory reactions.

Remodeling – the rebuilding of the skeleton, regulated by osteoblasts—cells that build up the skeleton, and osteoclasts—cells that break down the skeleton.

Renin-Angiotensin System (RAS) – a hormone system that regulates blood pressure and fluid and electrolyte balance, as well as systemic vascular resistance – blood pressure and blood flow.

Superoxide Anion Production – A superoxide is a compound that contains the superoxide ion. An anion is a negatively charged ion. The systematic name of the anion is "dioxide." The reactive oxygen ion superoxide is important as the product of the one-electron reduction of dioxygen (having two atoms of oxygen in the molecule).

Systolic blood pressure – the pressure of the blood in the arteries when the heart pumps. It is the higher of two blood pressure measurements.

Vitamin D Receptors (VDR) – bind to hormones and DNA proteins to affect gene expression and vitamin D synthesis. Also called calcitriol receptors, aid in vitamin D absorption and production, while helping to regulate vitamin D.

Vitamin D Deficiency – a serum 25-hydroxyvitamin D level less than 20 nanograms per milliliter (less than 50 nanomoles per liter).

Vitamin D Insufficiency – a serum 25-hydroxyvitamin D level of 20 to 30 nanograms per milliliter (50 to 75 nanomoles per liter).

Vascular Endothelial Dysfunction – a systemic pathological state of the endothelium.

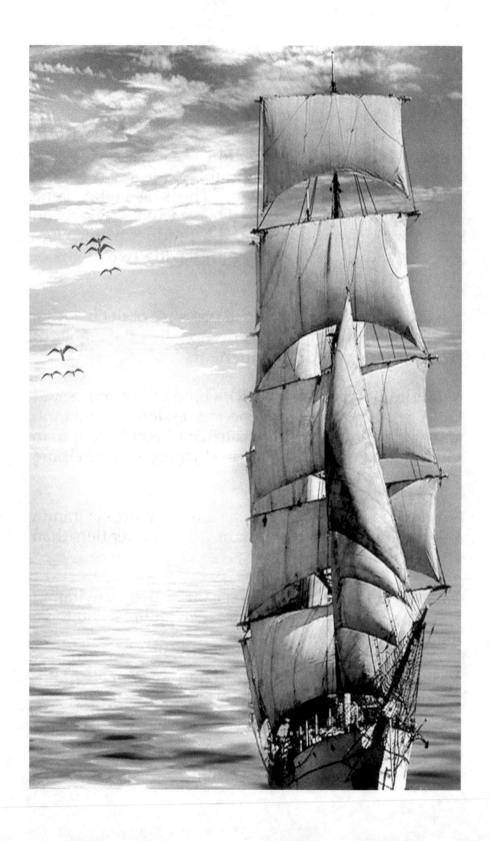

References & Resources:

https://www.ncbi.nlm.nih.gov/pmc/articles/PMC3593520/

https://www.ncbi.nlm.nih.gov/pmc/articles/PMC4153851/

https://www.eatingdisorderhope.com/blog/anorexia-bone-density-vitamin-d

https://www.ncbi.nlm.nih.gov/pubmed/28217829

https://www.easy-immune-health.com/vitamin-d-therapy.html

https://www.ncbi.nlm.nih.gov/pmc/articles/PMC3899558/

https://www.ncbi.nlm.nih.gov/pmc/articles/PMC5990512/

https://www.everydayhealth.com/arthritis/arthritis-and-vitamin-d-whats-the-connection.aspx

https://www.ncbi.nlm.nih.gov/pmc/articles/PMC3539179/

https://rheumatology.medicinematters.com/osteoarthritis-/diet-and-nutrition/vitamin-d-has-potential-benefits-for-people-with-osteoarthritis-/16929090

https://www.medicalnewstoday.com/articles/319617

https://www.uspharmacist.com/article/vitamin-d-and-chronic-pain-promising-correlates

https://paulingblog.wordpress.com/2011/06/15/casimir-funk-and-a-century-of-vitamins/

https://en.wikipedia.org/wiki/Vitamin_D

https://www.easy-immune-health.com/is-it-vit-d-deficiency-or-hypoglycemia.html

www.easy-immune-health.com/Vitamin-D-facts

https://www.grassrootshealth.net/project/daction/

https://drsircus.com/cancer/vitamin-d-deficiency-as-a-cause-of-diseases-safe-high-dose-vitamin-d-treatments/

https://ajph.aphapublications.org/doi/full/10.2105/AJPH.2004.045260

Vitamins in the Prevention of Human Diseases

https://www.cidrap.umn.edu/news-perspective/2020/04/new-york-obesity-appears-raise-covid-19-risk

https://www.frontiersin.org/articles/10.3389/fendo.2019.00103/full

https://www.diabetes.co.uk/food/vitamin-d.html

https://www.webmd.com/urinary-incontinence-oab/news/20100322/low-vitamin-d-linked-incontinence

https://www.ncbi.nlm.nih.gov/pmc/articles/PMC5491340/

https://www.webmd.com/lung/copd/news/20190111/is-daily-vitamin-d-a-lifesaver-for-copd-patients *https://spectrum.diabetesjournals.org/content/24/2/113*

https://www.ncbi.nlm.nih.gov/pubmed/29911760

https://www.ncbi.nlm.nih.gov/pmc/articles/PMC6013996/

https://www.ncbi.nlm.nih.gov/pmc/articles/PMC5743852/

https://www.ncbi.nlm.nih.gov/pmc/articles/PMC5691736/

https://www.healthgrades.com/right-care/migraine-and-headache/could-vitamin-d-cure-migraines

Clinical Infectious Diseases

https://clinicaltrials.gov/ct2/show/NCT04344041

https://www.sciencedaily.com/releases/2019/02/190206200347.htm

https://www.ncbi.nlm.nih.gov/pmc/articles/PMC3026680/

https://www.ncbi.nlm.nih.gov/pmc/articles/PMC4101586/

https://www.medicalnewstoday.com/articles/323919

https://link.springer.com/article/10.1007%2 Fs10067-010-1478-3

www.ncbi.nlm.nih.gov/pmc/articles/PMC5834596/

https://www.acam.org/blogpost/1092863/185723/Vitamin-D-Deficiency-and-Tooth-Decay

https://www.ncbi.nlm.nih.gov/pubmed/8140930

https://www.ncbi.nlm.nih.gov/pmc/articles/PMC5842009/

https://www.sciencedaily.com/ releases/2011/04/110403205232.htm

https://www.express.co.uk/life-style/health/1188900/ vitamin-d-deficiency-symptoms-dizziness-vertigo-causes-foods-treatment-supplements

https://www.ncbi.nlm.nih.gov/pmc/articles/PMC3897595/

https://advancedtissue.com/2014/11/vitamin-d-healing-wounds/

https://www.easy-immune-health.com/signs-of-magnesium-deficiency.html

https://drsircus.com/general/dosages-and-treatments-for-coronavirus-infections/

https://www.sciencedaily.com/ releases/2018/02/180226122548.htm

https://www.ncbi.nlm.nih.gov/pmc/articles/PMC4566462/

The Miraculous Cure for and Prevention of All Diseases, by Jeff T. Bowles

The Disease Conspiracy, Robert Barefoot

* * *

IMPORTANT NOTE:

If you think you may have a medical emergency, call your local emergency number immediately.

This information is not a substitute for professional medical advice, examination, diagnosis, or treatment. Do not delay or forego seeking treatment for a medical condition or disregard professional medical advice. Seek the advice of your physician, homeopath, naturopath, or other qualified healthcare professional before starting or changing any treatment.

* * *

About the Author

I live in a forest with a few domestic and numerous wild creatures, where I create an ever-growing inventory of books, both nonfiction and fiction, short stories, illustrated kid's books, and articles, with a bit of wood carving when I need a change of pace.

I received my Doctorate from the University of California at Irvine in the School of Social Sciences, majoring in psychology and ethnography, after which I moved to the Pacific Northwest to write and to have a modest private psychotherapy practice in a small town not much bigger than a village. Finally I decided it was time to put my full focus on my writing, where, through the world-shrinking internet, I could "meet" greater numbers of people. Where I could meet you!

All the creatures in my forest and I thank you for "stopping by." If *Save Your Life with the Dynamic Duo D3 and K2* has touched you in a positive way I hope you'll consider writing a review, as reviews are an excellent means for other people to discover books that might inspire them on their way.

If you would like to write to me, I'd love to hear from you – email below.

I Wish You Happiness, Health, Peace, and Joy,
Blythe

Blythe@BlytheAyne.com

www.BlytheAyne.com

CPSIA information can be obtained
at www.ICGtesting.com
Printed in the USA
LVHW080401201222
735602LV00004B/53

9 781947 151826